PPPD

A PATIENT'S GUIDE TO UNDERSTANDING
PERSISTENT POSTURAL-PERCEPTUAL DIZZINESS

PPPD

A PATIENT'S GUIDE TO UNDERSTANDING
PERSISTENT POSTURAL-PERCEPTUAL DIZZINESS

Mark Knoblauch PhD

Kiremma Press
Houston, TX

© 2019 by Mark Knoblauch

Printed in the United States of America

Disclaimer: The information provided within this book is for general informational purposes only. It is not intended to be a substitute for medical advice. While we try to keep the information up-to-date and correct, there are no representations or warranties, express or implied, about the completeness, accuracy, reliability, suitability or availability with respect to the information contained in this book for any purpose. Any use of this information is at your own risk. Furthermore, the methods described within this book are the author's personal thoughts and opinions. As such, they are not intended to be a definitive set of instructions for you to follow precisely. You may discover there are other methods and materials to accomplish the same end result.

www.authorMK.com

ISBN: 978-1-7333210-0-6

For those who understand the hidden misery and frustration of living with a chronic vestibular disorder

Table of Contents

Introduction

Annoying. Aggravating. Debilitating. For those who live every day with a vestibular disorder, such words could certainly be used to describe daily life. Whether it's the periodic vertigo that accompanies benign paroxysmal positional vertigo (BPPV) or the lingering headaches and unsteadiness associated with vestibular migraine, few understand the impact of a vestibular disorder until they actually have one. Only then do they understand the frustration that comes with cancelling plans at the last minute or the constant fear of a fall or an attack that can come without warning. Certainly, life with a vestibular condition can require significant adjustment.

In the past few years, the condition known as persistent postural-perceptual dizziness, or *PPPD*, has entered the vestibular scene. The official recognition of PPPD has given hope to people who suffer from the unique set of conditions that have previously not fit into any of the other dizziness-related diagnoses. Because it is so new on the vestibular scene, PPPD unfortunately does not have the extensive research library filled with prevalence and incidence rates or successful treatment protocols that have been afforded to many of the existing vestibular conditions such as Ménière's disease or vestibular migraine. Rather, the data and research that is focused on PPPD is still in its early phases of development, as what we largely know about the disease has been pulled from several other related medical conditions that are now collectively known as PPPD. Only now, with an official diagnosis having been established, can researchers direct their efforts specifically towards the condition of PPPD. As this directed effort continues, we should expect an improved understanding of PPPD as well as more focused treatment directives aimed at reducing the symptoms of PPPD and perhaps even eradicating its effects.

This book is designed to outline for you the patient what we currently know about PPPD, so as to provide you a comprehensive source to understand aspects such as who is affected, what the common symptoms are, how it is diagnosed, and how PPPD can affect your quality of life. As a person affected by several vestibular conditions myself, I understand well the frustration of not having a beneficial source of information about a specific medical condition. I remember the days of scouring the internet back when my symptoms started, trying to find quality information, only to discover that most of the information was based on personal opinion or was trying to draw me in toward buying some 'miracle cure'. Knowing how incapacitating my own life with a vestibular condition could be, I set out to write medical guidebooks that take the relevant research and condense it into a readable, easy-to-understand format that outlines the most pertinent information that patients need. And that is what I hope this book brings you – the information you want specific to PPPD, presented in a way that you can understand. This will in turn make you a more informed and empowered patient, allowing you to have directed and focused conversations with your medical provider as well as those around you.

To accomplish the goal of making you a more informed PPPD patient, we will start out by looking at the inner ear, a likely source of many of the symptoms associated with PPPD. We will outline the relevant anatomy of the vestibular system along with the physiology of how our balance and motion detection systems work. Next we will take an in-depth look at the symptom of dizziness, as dizziness itself is a nearly constant complaint among PPPD patients. We'll then focus on the condition of PPPD itself by looking at aspects such as incidence and prevalence rates, the common symptoms associated with PPPD, suspected causes, and the psychological side of PPPD. Then we'll walk through how the diagnosis of PPPD is made, including a thorough overview of the diagnostic criteria that have recently been established. We'll follow that with a look at the normal treatment plan for PPPD and several dizziness-related conditions, followed by a chapter in which I outline my own dealings with ongoing symptoms that closely resemble what patients experience with PPPD. We'll then end with a chapter that outlines several medical conditions that closely mimic the presentation of PPPD.

When diagnosed with a chronic vestibular disorder, there are often so many questions that patients want answers for. While this book will not likely answer every question you may have, it is hoped that the information contained within this book will provide you a solid foundation for understanding a bit more about the miserable condition of PPPD and also empower you with a set of facts and information that you can use to tackle the challenge of dealing with PPPD every day.

Now, let's get started on your journey of learning the intricacies of PPPD.

Chapter 1: The Vestibular System

WHILE IT MIGHT BE of interest to dive right into the intricacies of PPPD, I think it better that we first outline the underlying anatomy and physiology involved with this condition. In doing so, it can help provide you a relevant background that can serve as a foundation for the upcoming chapter that specifically targets what PPPD is and how it affects patients. In using this chapter to understand the anatomy that is likely associated with PPPD, you will be able to later visualize the affected structures and also be able to differentiate many of the associated components of the inner ear. So while this chapter may seem somewhat like an anatomy book at times, its real purpose is to provide you a solid foundation specific to both the anatomy involved with PPPD itself as well as provide an overview of those structures that have can influence balance, dizziness, and vertigo.

The rationale for being all-inclusive with the anatomy of the ear is that when these balance-related structures are functioning incorrectly, we are left with what ends up being some of the symptoms of PPPD: imbalance, dizziness, and possibly vertigo. Therefore, this chapter will highlight not only the major components of our inner ear but also outline how several of these structures are responsible for our ability to maintain balance and equilibrium.

Sections of the ear

Outer ear

The most noticeable component of what we commonly characterize as our 'ear' is the portion that we can see (Figure 1.1). This includes the large pinna as well as the ear canal that leads to the eardrum, which collectively makes up our outer ear. The function of the outer ear is largely limited to funneling sound into the eardrum, and as it is located well away from the inner ear structures that are likely involved with PPPD, the outer ear is not considered to have any involvement with the symptoms associated with PPPD.

Middle ear

The middle ear is the air-filled portion of the ear located behind the eardrum and housed within the temporal bone (Figure 1.1). This portion of the ear holds the three small bones – the malleus, stapes, and incus – that transfer sound from the eardrum to the inner ear. The most association you will likely have with the middle

18

ear is when you suffer the effects of an ear infection. As the middle ear is really nothing more than a space within the temporal bone, it too has no real involvement with PPPD.

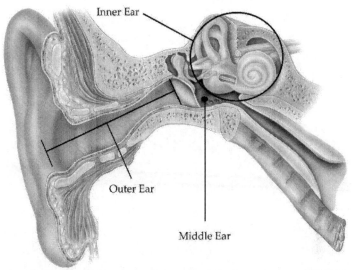

Figure 1.1. The three sections of the ear include the outer ear, middle ear, and inner ear. Issues involved with PPPD influence signals that are sent from the labyrinth portion of the inner ear

Inner ear

The inner ear is responsible for two major roles in our body. First, it detects and converts sound waves to neural impulses. In other words, it is responsible for our sense of hearing. While this is certainly no small feat, the inner ear is also responsible for the perception and interpretation of body positioning. This in turn makes the inner ear the site of both our main balance organ and our primary hearing organ.

Because of the intricate roles it has specific to hearing and motion detection, the inner ear is comprised of an array of highly sensitive structures. Unfortunately, the sensitivity of these structures also makes the inner ear quite susceptible to injury. Despite its small size, intricate structure, and dual responsibility for handling detection of both sound and motion, damage to the sensitive components of the inner ear can affect aspects that range from hearing to equilibrium. Furthermore, even minor disruptive events can trigger several symptoms such as motion sickness, vertigo, or nausea. Because of the high level of involvement of the inner ear structures in detecting sound and motion, the inner ear has been called one of the most intensively studied areas of vertebrate anatomy and physiology[1].

There are two main areas that make up the inner ear – the cochlea and the vestibular system. Together, these two structures make up what is known as the *labyrinth*. Despite what you often see in images of the inner ear, the labyrinth organs are not free-standing structures; rather, they are simply tunnels that exist deep within the temporal bone (Figure 1.2). These tunnels contain membranes that serve to contain the unique fluid (i.e. 'endolymph') contained within the labyrinth. As we will discuss, it is the movement of this fluid within the vestibular system that provides much of our ability to detect certain motions of the head.

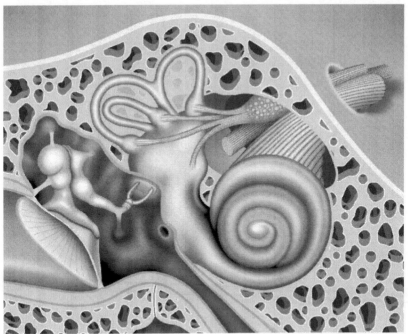

Figure 1.2 The labyrinth system does not consist of free-standing structures but rather a group of hollowed-out areas of the temporal bone that form a series of cavities and tunnels

The vestibular system

Although the inner ear isn't specifically implicated in PPPD, many of its components are thought to play a role in the associated symptoms of PPPD such as dizziness. Therefore, we will take a detailed look at the structure and function of these vestibular components thought to play a role in the symptoms associated with PPPD.

There are two primary systems at play within the inner ear (Figure 1.3). The first is the cochlea, a snail-shaped organ designed to convert sound waves to electrical signals that can be interpreted by the brain as 'sound'. Because there is not a common association between hearing loss and PPPD, there is relatively little direct involvement between PPPD and the cochlea. As such, in this chapter we'll focus predominantly on the vestibular system given its strong link to the symptoms that commonly occur in response to PPPD.

In terms of an overall purpose, the vestibular system of the inner ear has a primary role of detecting motion of the head, along with serving to provide feedback specific to an individual's head position. It is known that some structures of the vestibular system are involved in PPPD, and as a result we will take a comprehensive look at the components of the vestibular system in order to outline how aspects such as unsteadiness or vertigo – both commonly associated with PPPD – may develop. To do this, we first need to detail the anatomy of our vestibular system as well as the physiology of how these structures work to provide feedback specific to our head's movement and position.

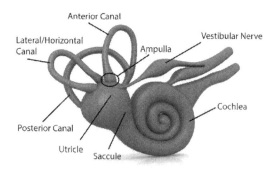

Figure 1.3. The labyrinth system is comprised of several individual organs including the cochlea, vestibule, and semicircular canals.

Vestibular anatomy

Five independent structures are involved in our ability to detect motion. The first two structures are housed within an organ termed the vestibule, a 3-5mm wide structure located between the cochlea and semicircular canals. The vestibule itself contains two very important components called the *saccule* and the *utricle* that are responsible for detecting motion that occurs in a linear direction (i.e. forward/backward, up/down, side-to-side). Activities such as running, walking, standing up, or even riding in an elevator are detected by the saccule and the utricle, and as we will discuss, both structures have thousands of small crystals embedded within them to help detect inertia. It is this inertia and the resulting motion of the saccule and utricle that is then processed and interpreted by the brain as movement of the head. Because the saccule and utricle house these small crystals known as *otoliths*, the utricle and saccule are commonly known as the "otolith organs".

In addition to the saccule and utricle, the remainder of the vestibular portion of the inner ear is comprised of three tunnels called semicircular canals that form loops through the temporal bone. These canals detect circular motion, the kind generated when you shake your head 'yes' or 'no'. The semicircular canals also play a very important role in ensuring that our eyes can stay on a fixed spot or target even while our head is moving, through a process we will discuss later in this chapter known as the vestibulo-ocular reflex. Without all of these structures functioning properly, our ability to maintain balance and have a normal equilibrium would be severely impaired. As we will outline, many of the symptoms of PPPD appear to result from some improperly functioning component of the vestibular system in that either the system itself is not working or some aspect is excessively sensitive to motion. To help clarify how all of these components interact to work as a functioning unit, we will next take a look at the structures of the vestibular system as well as outline how they work in helping us to detect movement and maintain equilibrium.

Saccule

The saccule is a structure within the vestibule that is responsible for detecting vertical motion of the head (and with movement of the head typically comes movement of the body as well). For example, jumping up and down or riding in an elevator are activities that stimulate the motion sensors within the saccule. Inside the saccule is a structure called the *macula sacculi*, a vertically-oriented organ which houses a two- to three-millimeter area comprised of sensory hair cells responsible for detecting head motion. The ends of these hair cells extend horizontally into the middle of the vestibule and are covered by a gelatinous layer, over which is a fibrous structure called the otolithic membrane

24

(Figure 1.4). This otolithic membrane is embedded with thousands of calcium-based crystals known by a variety of names including *statoconia, otoconia,* and the aforementioned *otolith*. For the purpose of this book we will use the term *otolith* to describe the crystals of the inner ear.

Because it is embedded with otoliths, the otolithic membrane is heavier than the material surrounding it.

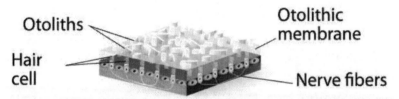

Figure 1.4 Otoliths embedded within the otolithic membrane activate hair cells in response to directional head motion (image is of the orientation of the macula utriculi)

Therefore, when the body moves somewhat quickly in a vertical plane such as occurs when jumping, gravity pulls the otoliths downward the same way as a leafy branch might bend when you swing it upward. The weight of the otoliths causes nerve cells that extend into the otolithic membrane to bend in response to the linear motion. This in turn causes those hair cells to send a signal to the brain that is interpreted as vertical movement of the head.

Utricle

The utricle has an almost identical makeup as the saccule but has a slightly different orientation and function. The utricle is larger than the saccule and operates by detecting when the head moves in the horizontal plane. Such movements, which occur with forward, backward, or side-to-side motion of the head, happen with walking, running, or even riding in a car. Like the saccule, the utricle contains a macula called the *macula utriculi*. In contrast to the saccule's vertically-oriented macula, the macula utriculi is positioned horizontally and is embedded with hair cells that are oriented vertically. The mechanism by which the macula utriculi detects motion operates similarly to that of the macula sacculi in that the hair cells are covered with a gelatinous layer which is in turn overlaid with a gel-like membrane embedded with otoliths.

Similar to the vertical action within the saccule, when forward, backward, or side-to-side head motion occurs within the utricle, the inertia created from the force of the motion upon the embedded otoliths creates a sort of 'shearing' motion between the gelatinous layer and the otolithic membrane. This motion is then detected by the utricle's embedded nerve cells which in turn send a signal to the brain that gets interpreted as a specific horizontal movement of the head.

Semicircular Canals

In addition to the vestibule's saccule and utricle structures, there are three semicircular canals of the inner ear's labyrinth network that make up the remainder of the vestibular system. As mentioned earlier, the semicircular canals are not true bony structures themselves; rather, they exist as 'tunnels' or canals through the temporal bone. Thin membranes line the bone-encased semicircular canals and serve to contain the fluid known as endolymph that is found throughout the labyrinth system. Like each maculi of the utricle and saccule that detect linear movement, rotational or 'angular' motions of the head cause this endolymph to move within the canals – a process that we will discuss shortly. An example of angular motion would include turning the head side-to-side as if watching a tennis match. Because this movement does not generate enough inertia within the inner ear to act upon the saccule or utricle, the design of the semicircular canals allows them to detect this angular motion as the endolymph flows across specialized sensors within each canal. The brain then interprets the signal from these sensors to establish the direction of head movement.

There are three independent semicircular canals – the anterior, posterior, and horizontal canals. The arrangement of the three canals positions them at right angles to each other which in turn allows all head motions to be detected. This design can be imagined by thinking of a corner of a cube – each of the three sides of the cube represents a different plane of movement similar to how any angular movement of the head can be detected by one or more of the semicircular canals.

So how does movement of fluid within the semicircular canals actually result in the brain being able to detect the motion? It's quite a fascinating process (at least in my mind!), actually. Angular motion is detected due to endolymph passing over a specialized organ within each canal called the *cupula*. Movement of the head in an angular motion (i.e. shaking the head 'no', nodding the head, etc.) causes movement of endolymph, which in turn flows across hair cells that move in response to the flow of endolymph. These hair cells are located within the canal itself, at each end of the semicircular canal in a bulged-out area called the *ampulla* (see Figure 1.3). Hair cells within the ampulla contain the cupula, a gelatinous layer over the hair cells that extends across the width of the ampulla.

Let's look at this process in a little more detail. When a person moves his or her head, the endolymph moves within the semicircular canal in response to the head movement. As the fluid moves, it flows around the cupula (Figure 1.5). As the fluid motion of the endolymph pushes against the cupula, the cupula bends in response to the fluid moving over it. This causes hair

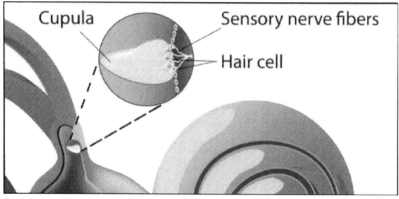

Figure 1.5. Near the end of each semicircular canal, the ampulla houses the sensitive cupula organ which is responsible for detecting movement of fluid within the respective semicircular canal

cells immediately under the cupula to also bend, the same way the aforementioned tree branch may bend if its leafy end were placed into flowing water. This bending of the hair cells sends a signal to the brain which is interpreted as motion appropriate to the direction of head movement.

These events occurring within the semicircular canals are important to understand, as they are largely thought to play a role in vertigo and dizziness. As far back as the 1960s, researchers believed that conditions such as benign paroxysmal positional vertigo (BPPV) – which triggers bouts of vertigo, nystagmus (rapid eye motion), and unsteadiness – resulted from otoliths pressing against the cupula within the semicircular canal[2]. This interference was suspected of increasing the cupula's sensitivity to motion, in turn generating the symptoms associated with BPPV.

Vertigo and the vestibular system

The preceding portion of this chapter has outlined in detail much about the vestibular system as well as relevant cranial nerves that we rely on for daily function. My reasoning for going into such detail with each is two-fold. First, I want you to have an understanding of the complexity of the vestibular system, for as we have discussed, this system is quite intricate. Even a small disruption to the vestibular system can have a significant impact on several aspects of our life. The extent of this impact leads to the second reason I wanted to outline the vestibular system in depth – to help you understand the mechanisms involved in balance and vertigo that can arise as a result of PPPD.

Vertigo is the sensation of movement when in fact no movement is occurring. It is important to understand that vertigo is a symptom – not an actual medical condition; therefore, expecting a cure for vertigo is effectively the same as expecting a cure for pain. What is likely meant is that one expects a cure for what is *causing* the vertigo. Vertigo itself is largely thought to result from events occurring within the inner ear, and other medical conditions that trigger vertigo – such as BPPV – are known to originate from within the inner ear. Still, other vertigo-inducing conditions such as PPPD are not as clear cut and are thought to involve a complex interaction between the brain (i.e. 'central' type vertigo) and the inner ear (i.e. 'peripheral' vertigo).

As a patient of a vestibular-related condition it is important to understand that vertigo has several possible sources, and no one event or structure has been established as a primary cause for vertigo. Researchers have largely narrowed peripheral vertigo down to the semicircular canals, saccule, or utricle, while central vertigo is typically associated with either the brainstem or the vestibulocochlear nerve[3]. When functioning normally, the inner ear structures send signals to the brain in a coordinated pattern from the left and right ear. However, an imbalance of these vestibular inputs – such as can occur when one of our two vestibular systems is not performing correctly – leads to uncoordinated information being transmitted to the brain, in turn triggering events such as nystagmus (rapid and uncontrollable eye movement) or vertigo to occur. This imbalanced signal can occur due to disruption anywhere along the neural pathway that stretches from the vestibular-based sensors to the brain.

Again, there is no specific structure or area that triggers vertigo across all patients. Therefore, vertigo can arise from multiple causes and conditions. For example, patients experiencing migraine (i.e. a specific type of headache) sometimes experience vertigo similar to patients who have a disorder specific to the vestibule of the inner ear. Sometimes vertigo even originates outside of the skull, such as can occur in patients who experience vertigo that results from degrading intervertebral discs, a condition known as 'cervical vertigo'[4].

One confounding issue that medical professionals have in establishing vertigo is that patients often lump it in with dizziness. Both vertigo and dizziness are indeed similar in their effects given that each can make you as the patient feel unsteady. One recommended way to separate the two conditions is to determine whether you feel 'lightheaded' or whether you feel as though the world is spinning around you. Generally, a spinning sensation is more characteristic of vertigo, while lightheadedness is typically associated with dizziness[5].

To reiterate, the symptom of vertigo occurs when the patient reports that their world is spinning around them despite the fact that they are stationary. So what exactly causes this sensation? Physiologically speaking, the sensation of vertigo is largely due to a link between

31

the inner ear and the eyes. While this may seem to be a somewhat odd link, the interconnection between our ears and eyes plays a vital role in our daily function even though we may not recognize it (until there is a problem!). To outline this role, we need to discuss the vestibulo-ocular reflex (VOR) and how it coordinates the interaction between the ear and eye.

The vestibulo-ocular reflex (VOR)

Although our eyes have independent functions specific to providing our sense of vision, they are intimately connected with the inner ear. This interaction plays an important role in our ability to maintain balance as well as to maintain visual acuity when we are moving. To see how important your vision is for aiding in your balance, walk quickly from a bright room into a very dark one. You'll probably find that you are initially timid and a little bit unsteady, which will likely improve once your eyes adjust to the darkness. Similarly, jump up and down a few times and notice how your vision of the field around you is still quite clear and steady – a stark contrast from watching a video that was recorded on a camera you held while jumping. The ability to maintain this smooth field of vision even while engaged in strenuous activity such as jumping is because of the intricate link between the vestibular system and the eyes. In fact, this link has even been given a name – the 'vestibulo-ocular reflex' (VOR). We won't go deep into the details of how the VOR works, but we will next provide a general overview of the reflex as it relates to a few expected symptoms of PPPD.

The interconnection between your vestibular system and eyes is what allows you to maintain a smooth, non-jumpy field of vision while running or riding on a bumpy road. This happens because the vestibular system actually has some control over the muscle of the eyes through the VOR that allows the eyes to remain fixed on an object even though one's head position may be moving. This reflex has the task of trying to ensure that an image or object remains stable on an individual's retina in order to allow for proper processing by the brain[6]. Without the VOR, every time your head moves, you would consciously need to readjust your eye position back to the object you are looking at. With the VOR, however, your vestibular system is able to detect the speed of your head motion and automatically control the muscles in your eye so that your gaze easily remains fixed on the object. This reflex also works well when driving, as every time you hit a bump or turn a corner your eyes are subconsciously controlled by the VOR rather than jumping all around while trying to manually reposition – which would certainly be a problem when operating a vehicle!

When the VOR is working correctly you don't even know that it's there. But when there is a disruption to the system – such as occurs in response to a vestibular-related disease such as PPPD – the VOR becomes impaired and can lead to uncontrolled movements such as the aforementioned nystagmus or the spinning sensation associated with vertigo. Consequently, an affected patient is not able to coordinate their eye movements with the movements of their head. This can lead to jumpy or blurry vision, likely occurring most often when the head is moving or the patient's body is in motion. Another condition that can result is *oscillopsia,* a condition in which objects in the field of vision appear to float around even though they are in fact stationary, due in large part to the muscles of the eye being unable to keep the eye adequately fixed on one object.

Additional problems occur when a person with a faulty VOR tries to follow movement or read text on paper or a computer screen, an event known as *tracking*. With the VOR not allowing for smooth eye movement such as that required to follow a thrown ball or read printed text, it can be difficult for the patient to make the precise eye motions needed to properly intake visual information (i.e. identify and process the written words). Without a well-established link between our eyes and our ears, life would be much more difficult. But unfortunately, because of this link between our eyes and ears we must often pay the price of having visual disturbances such as vertigo or nystagmus any time our vestibular system is malfunctioning.

Conclusion

Clearly, the inner ear consists of highly intricate and complex structures that are vital for our normal function. Without a properly functioning vestibular system, our ability to maintain posture, recognize our movements, and sense positional changes can be extremely difficult. The intent of this chapter was to provide an overview of those structural components of the inner ear involved in PPPD. In addition, we touched on several physiological processes that can occur in response to PPPD such as vertigo. Understand that what we covered in this chapter is indeed quite generic in scope; there is in fact much, much more that we could discuss at a much deeper level. However, as I stated in the introduction, my focus is to keep this book oriented as a guide for PPPD patients rather than serving as a medical textbook. What you will hopefully find is that as you read through this book, the detailed information we have discussed here becomes more relevant to you given that you now better understand the various anatomy and physiology of the inner ear. But first, we'll take a detailed look in the next chapter at dizziness, one of the most prevalent factors associated with PPPD and a symptom that has significant effects along with many potential causes. In understanding the various sources of dizziness along with the events that cause dizziness symptoms, you as the patient of a dizziness-related condition can more easily understand just what dizziness is, as well as the likely factors responsible for triggering dizziness episodes.

Chapter 2: Dizziness

UNDERSTANDING THE VESTIBULAR system is key to being able to recognize the underlying structures and physiology involved in PPPD. While imbalance and vertigo are common complaints of PPPD, these symptoms can somewhat be accounted for with an understanding the physiology of the inner ear's vestibular system. Dizziness, however, is another symptom of PPPD that is a bit more complicated as to its origins despite it being a relatively common condition even in otherwise healthy people. Therefore, this chapter will focus on outlining just what dizziness is as well discussing the many potential causes of dizziness. In understanding the causes of dizziness, it can help patients separate out PPPD-related dizziness from the many other potential causes.

What is dizziness?

Dizziness is a symptom, much like pain. And it can be a costly symptom, with current medical expense estimates of up to $50 billion per year resulting from dizziness[7]. Because dizziness is a symptom which must be reported and described by the patient, we do not have a good test which can measure the type or degree of dizziness that a patient experiences[8]. Whereas there are no tests for dizziness, patients are often required to describe their dizziness, which can be difficult for a patient to do[9]. It is also important to separate dizziness from vertigo. Vertigo is the perception of movement when no movement is actually occurring. If you've ever had vertigo, you are familiar with the sensation that seems as though the room is spinning, or that you are spinning within the room. Dizziness is not vertigo, though, and does not involve perceived motion as much as a sensation that one's balance is 'off' or that they feel lightheaded.

Much like pain, dizziness can come in many forms and can be the result of many different causes. It is relatively common, with up to 8% of people reporting dizziness at some point in their lifetime[10]. Unfortunately, dizziness does not have a clear definition[11], likely because dizziness comes in many forms in much the same way that pain has many potential forms. For example, pain can be achy, or sharp, or dull and can arise from a joint, bone, nerve impingement, or tissue trauma, amongst others. Likewise, dizziness can result from positional changes (e.g. going around a corner), standing up from a seated position, low blood pressure, or even from an ear infection. Still, it is expected that a patient complaining of dizziness generally has some sort of issue that affects their posture and or gait[8]. Recognizing the various causes as well as effects of dizziness can help differentiate the dizziness associated with PPPD from the many other forms.

Causes of dizziness

As mentioned, 'dizziness' as a symptom can come in many forms. Some of the various conditions that could be intermixed with the general understanding of the term 'dizziness' could include nausea, vertigo, lightheadedness, imbalance, or unsteadiness[11]. Because of these various causes, up to 35% of the population is said to experience some degree of dizziness during their life[12], and is one of the most common reasons for visits to a physician[13]. Furthermore, up to 12% of people in the United States are thought to have experienced dizziness in the past 12 months[14], and the percent of people affected get much higher in an older population[12]. However, it's also known that up to half of individuals who report dizziness do not seek medical attention[15], suggesting that the actual number of people who experience dizziness is much higher.

Dizziness associated with the vestibular system typically influences a patient's sense of balance when moving his or her head[11]. In fact, some of the most common causes of dizziness that resulted in a medical evaluation are localized to the inner ear, as one study reported that BPPV was the most common cause (33.9%), phobic postural vertigo was next (21.4%), followed by Ménière's disease (20%), vestibular neuronitis/labyrinthitis (8.1%), and vestibular migraine (4.1%)[13]. When dizziness is of a vestibular source, the issue typically lies with one or both balance organs (e.g. semicircular canals, vestibule), the vestibular nerve that carries the signal from the balance organs to the brain, or the brain's ability to process the signals[16]. Initially, a significant degree of vertigo or imbalance will occur in response to diminished function of a vestibular organ until the brain adequately adjusts to the diminished function, including during those times that the patient is not moving[16]. Hours or days later, the patient will likely have a much lower degree of symptoms when stationary, but will begin to or continue to have similar issues when movement occurs. Overcoming this phase of vestibular deficit takes longer and often requires specific exercises to help the brain adapt to the diminished vestibular function[16]. In addition, a patient will likely have a smoother recovery if the dizziness only occurs in one ear[16]. If both inner-ear vestibular mechanisms are compromised, recovery will take longer and the patient will most likely experience symptoms even during normal activity[16].

Vestibular issues are not the only cause for dizziness, as patients who feel imbalance after moving to a standing position may have cardiac or circulatory issues rather than a vestibular-based source of dizziness. For example, dizziness can occur in patients with low blood pressure who cannot maintain adequate blood flow to the brain when moving from a lying or seated position to standing[17]. Other instances include dizziness that occurs when the eyes are moved in absence of head movement, which suggests an anxiety-related source[11]. Because PPPD is largely related to dizziness of a vestibular origin, we will not discuss these cardiac or anxiety-related causes.

Impact of dizziness

It's one thing to have dizziness, but it's another issue if the dizziness affects an individual's daily life. One study reported that their dizziness affected patients' daily activities, caused them to avoid leaving the house, and even required sick leave from work[15]. This in turn results in an impact on an individual's quality of life, social life, and ability to perform normal daily tasks[12], which can invite feelings of helplessness as well as result in a patient isolating themselves from others. Furthermore, as dizziness is somewhat related to one's ability to maintain balance, experiencing dizziness can increase the risk of falls which in turn can cause injury and result in significant medical costs[18]. The injury and subsequent medical expense contribute heavily to the resulting decrease in quality of life that dizziness can bring[19].

Treatment of dizziness

To treat a patient's dizziness it is first essential to understand the source of the dizziness. For example, if a patient simply has an ear infection there is no benefit to giving them blood pressure medication as a means to improve their dizziness, as the ear infection is the true source. Therefore, a simple dose or two of antibiotics may indeed clear their dizziness symptoms within a day or two. If the cause of the dizziness is vestibular in nature, it is essential that the particular vestibular condition is identified. For example, if the patient is experiencing dizziness associated with BPPV, a relatively simple procedure can 'reset' the problematic cause of the dizziness. Other vestibular-related dizziness, such as Ménière's disease or vestibular neuritis, may be improved by lifestyle changes such as going on a low-sodium diet, undergoing balance training therapy, or may be improved through the use of certain prescription (e.g. triptans) or non-prescription (e.g. dimenhydrinate) drugs. Unfortunately, though, some vestibular-related dizziness does not respond well to treatment and may require adjustments on the part of the patient such as using assistance (e.g. cane) when walking or requiring transportation help.

Conclusion

Because ongoing dizziness is a major aspect of PPPD, I felt it was relevant to discuss the possible causes and impact of dizziness. If PPPD is a diagnosis you have received yourself, there is a very likely chance that you are experiencing vestibular-related dizziness rather than any type related to a cardiac source. Now that we have covered both the vestibular system and the symptom of dizziness, you have a firm overview toward understanding the mechanisms involved in PPPD. Therefore, we will next dive into PPPD as a medical condition itself, drawing on what we understand about the inner ear in order to help outline aspects such as the suspected cause, the symptoms, and who is affected.

Chapter 3 – What is PPPD?

PERSISTENT POSTURAL-PERCEPTUAL dizziness (PPPD) is a newly-recognized condition that is thought to be influenced by an interplay between the vestibular system and the brain. More specifically, PPPD is suspected to occur in response to a sort of 'disagreement' between what the inner ear's vestibular system detects and what the brain wants to believe about the person's body position or balance[20]. In general, patients affected by PPPD are afflicted with chronic vertigo as well as dizziness that is often made worse when the patient is put into certain positions or when certain visual stimuli are presented[21].

As a medical condition, PPPD is one of the newest recognized vestibular disorders, only publishing its official diagnostic criteria in 2017. As such, there is not a strong history in the medical literature that outlines the factors involved in PPPD like there is with other, more established vestibular conditions such as Ménière's disease or acoustic neuroma. However, given that PPPD is now recognized as a true medical condition, researchers have begun to focus more effort into outlining certain characteristics of the disease which in turn helps identify specific criteria associated with PPPD. In this chapter we will outline just what PPPD is – specific to who it affects, its suspected causes, and the common symptoms. In doing so, you will have a better understanding of just what PPPD is as a medical condition.

Evolution of the term PPPD

Prior to the official recognition of PPPD, symptoms associated with the disease were often classified as one of several other medical conditions. For example, *space and motion discomfort, psychogenic dizziness, phobic postural vertigo, chronic subjective dizziness, psychophysiological dizziness*[16] and *visual vertigo*[22] are all diseases that the symptoms of PPPD could fit into before being reclassifed as its own disease. Patients exhibiting the symptoms of this 'early form' of PPPD were often diagnosed with *chronic vestibulopathy* or *psychogenic dizziness*, each of which is no longer recommended[23]. Eventually, researchers came together and focused their attention towards recognizing many of the similar characteristics of these diseases. This eventually led to the official recognition of PPPD.

A background of PPPD

As a medical condition, PPPD has a very short history and – compared to other vestibular conditions – a scarcity of data that can be used to help outline factors associated with the disease. Because of the relatively short history of PPPD, and because of the overlap in symptoms that PPPD shares with other vestibular disorders, I thought that it would be beneficial to take a moment to look at the medical progression used for establishing PPPD as an independent condition.

As far back as the late 1800s scientists recorded events of dizziness in response to high-motion environments[24]. Later, researchers established certain underlying situations (e.g. postural control, threat assessment) that characterized what became known as "fear of the marketplace"[25]. Physicians also began to piece together that certain underlying inner-ear conditions could worsen *agoraphobia* (fear of places that could trigger a panic attack), particularly in people with existing anxiety[26].

Much debate existed among researchers as to whether the events involved in these situations were neurologic in nature or psychiatric[23]. As the field of psychology grew, agoraphobia became associated more with psychology than with the inner ear[23], while the potential link with inner-ear involvement was largely forgotten[23, 27]. Fast-forward to the 1980s, and medicine again began to focus on the potential link between the inner ear and anxiety. In 1986, phobic postural vertigo (PPV) was recognized as a medical condition involving postural dizziness and bouts of unsteadiness along with mild anxiety and depression in patients who had also been diagnosed with obsessive compulsory personality

47

traits[28]. Researchers recognized that PPV was relatively common and had a separate presentation from many of the other vestibular conditions known at the time, and that PPV seemed to develop from a 'miscommunication' of sorts between anticipated and actual physical movement[23]. This miscommunication in turn caused patients to adapt an altered posture in order to address the inherent miscommunication.

Around this same time, researchers began to focus on a set of patients who noted particular problems in response to movement when they were in what is known as "visually-rich environments". Situations such as riding in a car on a street lined with thin shadows, or walking down long hallways with a particular carpet pattern could cause a degree of uneasiness for these patients who were suffering from what was termed *space and motion discomfort* (SMD)[29]. Later, *visual vertigo* (VV) was diagnosed in certain patients who felt dizzy or unsteady when exposed to certain visual stimuli[30]. It was recognized that the triggers of VV closely resembled the known triggers for SMD[31], with researchers eventually determining that patients of VV often exhibited a heightened awareness of potential vestibular symptoms in addition to being more reliant on visual input to establish their own spatial orientation[32].

In the early 2000s, a condition called *chronic subjective dizziness* (CSD) was recognized that was very similar to PPV yet highlighted the physical components of the condition rather than the psychological aspects. And, a diagnosis of CSD required dizziness – not vertigo

– along with symptoms of unsteadiness, a heightened sensitivity to motion, and difficulty in doing tasks that required a precise visual focus[33].

With the advent of CSD, and given its similarity to other dizziness-related conditions, it can become increasingly difficult to correctly classify a patient into one diagnosis or another as it is rare that a patient's symptoms fit perfectly into one category. Still, in 2010, the Committee for Classification of Vestibular Disorders of the Barany Society began to investigate the research surrounding PPV, CSD, space motion discomfort, and visual vertigo in order to determine if a larger, more inclusive medical condition was actually present[34]. From their work, the group was able to identify one higher-level condition that eventually became known as PPPD.

One of the benefits of combining these multiple diseases into one new medical condition is that the research involved with each of the preceding conditions can be incorporated into the collective evidence used to better understand PPPD. So even though as a recognized disease PPPD is relatively 'young' amongst other vestibular disorders, the combined evidence gathered on the predecessors of PPPD is quite extensive.

Epidemiology

The field of epidemiology involves the study of how widespread a disease is along with outlining the characteristics of who is affected. One of the most common ways to study the reach of a particular disease is to look at its *incidence* and *prevalence.* These two areas involve how many new cases of a particular disease arise in a year ('incidence') as well as how many people are currently affected by a disease ('prevalence').

In the case of PPPD, its newness as a medical condition makes the determination of incidence and prevalence somewhat difficult because there are not years-worth of data to use in determination of incidence and prevalence[21]. So while there are no studies that have established the incidence or prevalence of PPPD[35], there are estimates available that are taken from other diseases that would have fallen into the realm of a PPPD diagnosis had the condition been established in the literature. These estimates are taken from patients with similar disease conditions such as phobic postural vertigo (PPV) or chronic subjective dizziness (CSD)[35]. Consequently, at this time the best information we have specific to prevalence for PPPD is that it occurs in around 15-20% of patients who are evaluated for vestibular conditions. Separately, 4% of patients who saw a general practitioner in the United Kingdom reported persistent dizziness, most of whom were largely incapacitated as a result of their symptoms[36]. And among dizziness clinics, phobic postural vertigo or chronic subjective dizziness make up around 15-20% of all patient conditions[34]. These values make PPPD the second most common vestibular condition among adults, trailing only benign paroxysmal positional vertigo (BPPV)[35], but the most common cause of chronic dizziness within neurotology evaluations[37].

Incidence, or the number of new cases that occur per year, is also quite poorly understood for PPPD. To the best of our knowledge, the most relevant estimates for incidence of PPPD are around 25% of all patients who reported acute or episodic vestibular disorders[35]. In other words, one-fourth of individuals with episodic or acute vertigo attacks fall into the realm of PPPD. But again, because PPPD is so new as a medical condition it is tough to get an accurate set of data that provides specific incidence rates specific to PPPD rather than one of its preceding conditions. Therefore, as more cases are diagnosed as PPPD in the near future we will be better able to establish the true incidence of PPPD. Still, when monitoring individuals with other vestibular conditions such as BPPV, persistent dizziness consistent with what occurs in PPPD patients exists in around 1 out of 4 patients[35]. This suggests that the true incidence of PPPD may be much higher than originally thought, particularly among patients diagnosed with other vestibular disorders.

Besides incidence and prevalence rates, another important aspect of the epidemiology relates to the characteristics of the individuals who are affected. Such characteristics include aspects such as gender, age, etc. With PPPD, the evidence indicates that the average patient is in their mid-40s; however, a range of patient ages has been reported from the teenage years through late adulthood[35]. Though not clearly established in the medical literature, initial reports suggest that females have a slightly higher rate of PPPD than their male counterparts[35, 38].

Symptoms of PPPD

The symptoms of a disease relate to what the patient experiences in response to having that particular medical condition. Symptoms are subjective in nature; therefore, they cannot be measured with an existing piece of equipment and instead must be reported by the patient. For example, we cannot measure pain. We must instead rely on the patient to tell us how bad his or her pain is. While reporting one's pain can be beneficial to any medical professional, it also invites the problem that pain can be perceived differently for each patient. For example, one person may feel that a broken leg is a "4" out of a "10", while another person may rate the pain in their identical fracture as a "10". Consequently, symptoms such as pain or dizziness can vary quite significantly between individuals. This issue is further confounded by the fact that the patient's perspective of their symptoms – specific to intensity or degree of impairment – often conflicts with what the physician finds during evaluation[21]. Consequently, obtaining a diagnosis of PPPD can be a frustrating process for many patients.

In the world of PPPD, the majority of what patients experience as a result of the disease is largely symptom-related. And like most vestibular disorders, the symptoms associated with PPPD can be unique to each patient. In other words, symptoms are not always consistent from one patient to the next which in turn can add to the difficulty in diagnosing PPPD. For example, dizziness and vertigo are two common symptoms of PPPD, but we currently have no way to accurately and consistently measure dizziness or a patient's degree of vertigo. Therefore, medical professionals have to rely on what the patient reports in order to determine the degree and/or type of vertigo or dizziness that the patient is experiencing. As an example, the dizziness associated with PPPD might be characterized through a variety of descriptors that can include cloudiness, fuzziness, fullness, or lightheadedness, along with patients reporting that their visual focus is not clear[35]. Similarly, unsteadiness or certain types of vertigo are also highly associated with PPPD.

Further complicating the issue is that many other vestibular conditions can occur that exhibit very similar symptoms as PPPD[16]. Many of these conditions are much more established and popular in the medical literature, which might serve to inhibit a medical professional's ability to recognize the relatively new condition of PPPD over one of the more common vestibular disorders.

In addition to the varying symptoms between patients and its similarity to other vestibular conditions, it is important to point out that PPPD is considered a functional disorder rather than strictly a structural or psychiatric one[39]. This means that the symptoms associated with PPPD affect an individual's functional capacity but is not isolated to a particular structure in the ear or brain. One of the main symptom-based complaints of PPPD is some sort of vestibular impairment (e.g. dizziness, unsteadiness, etc.) throughout most every day[40]. When this impairment is not present, the span of time in which patients feel almost 'normal' is often only minutes or a few hours in length, though in rare cases, patients may note symptom-free phases that can last weeks[35]. Further evidence for the unique characteristics of PPPD are evident in the fact that some patients with certain other vestibular disorders often report a worsening of their symptoms when performing multiple activities such as talking while turning their head[16]. Patients with PPPD, however, seem to be distracted by such multitasking and often claim that their symptoms are suppressed in such situations.

Despite fluctuations in how PPPD presents itself, there are generally three main factors that tend to aggravate the degree of symptoms that PPPD patients experience. These factors include maintaining an upright posture, active or passive motion, or an exposure to moving visual activity or complex visual patterns. Now, let's take a look at each of these particular situations in more detail.

Upright posture

An upright posture tends to trigger symptoms to a greater degree in PPPD patients than when they are lying down[40]. In fact, reports indicate that standing or walking can even cause a greater degree of symptoms than sitting[35]. Lying down or at least in a recumbent position tends to reduce symptoms, even though the patient's symptoms are not likely resolved completely[35]. When upright, patients can attempt to reduce the effects of their symptoms through the use of walking aids, touching fixed objects, or holding on to another individual[35]. In many cases, even a light touch is reported to be enough to provide beneficial assistance.

Active or passive motion

Patients often report that active (the patient is moving him or herself) or passive (the patient is being transported, such as in a car) movement can worsen symptoms[35]. As the degree of motion increases, such as moving at a higher speed, the patient's symptoms tend to increase proportionally[35]. In fact, very high-speed movements seem to be the worst for provoking symptoms, regardless of whether the patient is actively or passively moving[35]. As the speed of movement decreases, there is more variability as to whether a patient will be affected or not[35]. Interestingly, some patients report that slower movements such as walking are actually preferable over remaining still[34].

Visual stimuli

Aggravation of PPPD symptoms in response to visual stimuli can occur from a variety of situations. In particular, 'busy' areas of visual stimuli appear to be problematic, such as being in large crowds, interacting in high-traffic areas, or even walking down a supermarket aisle[35]. Additionally, vast fields of vision can also trigger some patients as might occur with wide-open fields or large warehouse expanses[35]. Even a brief amount of time in such areas can cause hours or more of heightened symptoms for PPPD patients[35].

Some PPPD patients also report difficulty in using or focusing on very small visual points, particularly when held at a close range[35]. This reflects a similar issue of difficulty with computer use or watching television[35]. Given our society's high dependence on mobile and electronic devices, life with PPPD can be quite challenging for many patients.

In absence of such triggering conditions (e.g. visual motion, open expanses, computer use, etc.), symptoms can at times be quite minimal, often existing as a low but steady degree of chronic dizziness or unsteadiness. When symptoms are again triggered, patients report that significant unsteadiness along with vertigo are typically the most prominent[35].

Some of the recognizable aspects of PPPD occur as a result of the chronic dizziness that exists. As you have probably experienced yourself, a bout of dizziness typically generates a postural reaction in order to prevent or lessen the chance of falling. This reaction can include activity such as holding on to a sturdy object (e.g. handrail, chair, etc.) to prevent falling or might result in a reduction of head movement so as to lessen the degree of activity detected by the vestibular organs of the inner ear[16]. Similarly, avoidance of places where a fall could be particularly problematic (e.g. busy streets) as well as an increased awareness of potential tripping hazards can also occur[16]. This enhanced awareness of falls, as is inherent to PPPD patients, typically leads to a greater dependence upon visual input of a patient's environment rather than relying on vestibular input[16], even when the vestibular system is functioning normally.

Such compensations in aspects like postural adjustments or even gait patterns are common in PPPD patients[16], along with an increased awareness of the symptoms of dizziness[16]. In fact, certain personality traits such as neuroticism have been outlined as potential predecessors of PPPD[41]. Consequently, PPPD patients are constantly aware of their balance as they continually perform a sort of ongoing self-monitoring in order to try to prevent further vertigo attacks[41]. This constant awareness then leads in to the ever-present symptoms of PPPD such as a stiff posture, altered gait, and an increased use of visual stimuli to process one's balance[41].

Suspected cause of PPPD

At present there is no known cause for PPPD. Consequently, we are left with trying to establish a cause based upon the various signs and symptoms that patients commonly report. Given the relative 'newness' of PPPD, a verified cause may be elusive for at least the near future given that it can take years of testing and verification in order to establish a firm disease cause. However, as research continues to be conducted, every medical study contributes some small factor that can in turn provide valuable information. As these individual factors continue to build in number, trends can be established which in turn allow for directed, focused research toward establishing a true cause.

For most patients, PPPD begins after a specific vestibular incident such as vestibular neuritis or BPPV[41, 42]. In one study, the most common vestibular incident for initiating PPPD was reported to be vestibular neuritis, which caused almost 40% of PPPD diagnoses. Next up was BPPV, which caused just over 10%[43]. These findings are similar to other reports, as up to one-fourth of PPPD patients report some event such as BPPV or vestibular neuritis prior to their ongoing symptoms, while another 20% of patients report a preceding vestibular-based migraine attack[21]. However, a vestibular event is not required for initiating PPPD, as psychological events such as anxiety or a traumatic life event can also trigger PPPD[41]. In addition, head trauma has been noted as the triggering event in up to 15% of patients[21].

In many cases, the patient will recover from the initial inner-ear episode and have normal vestibular diagnostic tests, yet the patient will continue to have symptoms of dizziness[42]. As of yet, though, it remains unknown as to why some patients develop PPPD after a particular vestibular event[20]. Evidence suggests that there are changes within the brain among patients with PPPD. For example, a virtual reality roller coaster simulation revealed that PPPD patients showed decreased activity within certain areas of the brain during the simulation compared to healthy individuals[44]. Similarly, PPPD patients have been shown to have less grey matter in their brain than healthy controls, and those who have had the condition longer also showed lower levels of grey matter[45]. In addition, PPPD patients show decreased brain perfusion which can lead to problems with aspects such as mood and response inhibition[46]. Along with a few other (quite complicated) studies, the consensus remains that certain areas of the brain appear to be less active or may have less inter-connectivity in PPPD patients as compared to healthy individuals[41, 47].

As outlined earlier, PPPD patients seem to have a tendency to prefer or emphasize visual sensory input over vestibular-based input[47]. In other words, patients seem to want to suppress what their balance receptors are telling them about their body position (e.g. walking surface, head position, etc.) and instead tend to rely more on visual feedback in order to determine their body position. Similarly, patients who have sensory issues in areas such as their feet may not be able to transmit appropriate feedback from these areas[44], in turn leading to a greater disposition to rely on visual feedback. Furthermore, functional magnetic resonance imaging (MRI) has shown that PPPD patients exhibit reduced neural connectivity in the vestibular areas of the brain, thereby forcing them to rely more on visual inputs than healthy individuals[48].

It is also important to understand whether any medications could be the source of a patient's dizziness symptoms, which ultimately may be similar to those symptoms of PPPD. For example, some medications have side effects such as dizziness or unsteadiness, both of which can mimic the symptoms of PPPD[21]. Therefore, patients should be willing to inform their medical provider of all medications being taken so as to rule out any potential influence that the medication may be having on their symptoms[21].

The psychological side of PPPD

If you're reading this book as a person who has never had vertigo or severe dizziness, it can be difficult to understand the impact that either of these conditions can have on your daily life. A person who experiences vertigo commonly, however, can tell of the difficulty and/or frustration with seemingly menial tasks such as going to the store or keeping an appointment. The difficulty that dizziness and vertigo can bring also invite the psychological element that is involved with PPPD. Because fear or anxiety is an expected accompaniment to symptoms such as vertigo and dizziness, each must be accounted for in patients with PPPD[16]. In fact, patients with anxiety or certain other personality traits appear to be more susceptible to PPPD than those without[21]. One study reported that 60% of patients with PPPD met the criteria for an anxiety disorder[33], while a separate study found that two-thirds of patients with PPPD exhibited mood disorders and/or anxiety[49].

Experiencing the effects of PPPD can also generate a type of fear or anxiety in patients. For example, patients often begin to avoid busy places such as supermarkets or large events such as concerts. This behavior is similar to the aforementioned *agoraphobia,* or a fear of situations that could trigger a panic attack, but such an association is often incorrect in PPPD patients[20]. Rather, these types of settings have a high degree of visual stimulation which can be problematic for PPPD patients[20]. Other patients exhibit a fear of walking on smooth or very open surfaces[20], perhaps because there is not adequate visual or sensory feedback to provide them enough information as to the body position. Others have issues with driving on open roads – particularly when a certain speed is reached – to the point that patients have been known to purchase several cars prior to getting professional help[20]. These findings outline the clear fact that PPPD can warrant treatment on the psychological side of patient care as well as the physical.

One author put the psychological aspect of the fear and anxiety associated with PPPD into a unique perspective[20]. The human walking pattern is quite complex, and takes us approximately two years to master in our early life. Still, despite a general inability to walk, as infants and toddlers we had no fear of falling despite the fact that we fell almost every time we made our early walking attempts. As adults, however, our mastery of walking can be challenged in response to vestibular-related issues, in turn creating an immense fear of falling that had previously not existed. Therefore, we as vestibular patients attempt to control this fear by using a modified walking pattern and keeping a stiffened upper-body, and we often limit our head movement. Not unexpectedly, this is often the gait pattern observed in PPPD patients. Along these same psychological lines, research has shown that an individual's personal perception of life events also influences their susceptibility to PPPD. For example, patients who demonstrate *resilience* (i.e. the trait of being able to mentally recover from difficulty) had less persistent dizziness after a vestibular event[50]. In other words, patients who possessed the psychological ability to quickly move on from a troubling event reported less lingering dizziness. Similarly, individuals with a family history of anxiety were more likely to develop persistent dizziness[51]. Collectively, the evidence suggests that individuals who exhibit certain personality traits – or a family history of anxiety disorders – are at higher risk for developing PPPD[35]. Furthermore, having an introverted personality or neuroticism can also predispose an individual toward having PPPD[21, 52].

Understanding the cognitive model of panic disorder may help explain the psychological link behind PPPD. With panic disorder, patients experience repeated panic attacks as a result of misreading or misunderstanding the feedback they are receiving about body position and sensations[53]. This in turn causes a self-perpetuating response due to the fact that the misinterpretation of the feedback causes heightened anxiety which in turn leads to an increase in the misinterpreted feedback signal. In patients with vestibular disorders, the feedback is most likely originating from the balance detectors of the inner ear. Therefore, treatment which can help 'tone down' these misinterpreted signals – such as cognitive behavior therapy or vestibular rehabilitation – can be of great benefit to the patient.

Conclusion

The relative newness of PPPD as a medical condition leaves much to be discovered about what causes PPPD, what the symptoms represent, and who is most likely to be affected. Still, we do have other, related medical conditions that have provided some insight into the intricacies of PPPD. As the research continues to hone in on PPPD as a separate medical condition, we will learn more as to the underlying cause as well as the structures which are affected. And as we begin to narrow down the affected anatomy along with the physiological cause of PPPD we can begin to direct treatments toward specific areas of the body, with the hope of reversing the chronic instability and dizziness that PPPD brings. Next we will look at the diagnosis of PPPD specific to the criteria that must be met in order to separate PPPD from any of the other similar yet different dizziness-related conditions.

Chapter 4 – Diagnosis of PPPD

A COLLECTION OF SPECIFIC symptoms in a patient leads medical professionals to narrow down the most likely conditions that are causing those symptoms. Eventually, a diagnosis is reached that not only recognizes the official medical condition but also allows for a tailored treatment plan to be developed. Because PPPD is not only a newly recognized condition but also one that closely mimics other vestibular conditions, diagnosis can be somewhat difficult – particularly for those medical professionals who are not familiar with PPPD as a disease.

Many medical conditions, both vestibular in nature as well as non-vestibular, can cause significant and chronic dizziness. Consequently, any misdiagnosis can result in a failure to get relief from their symptoms simply because the appropriate treatment is not being applied to the correct condition or disease. With PPPD, it is recommended that a diagnosis is made by a specialist trained in vestibular disorders[16]. Such specialists include an ear, nose, and throat specialist, a neurologist, or an otoneurologist. Unfortunately, there is not an individual test that recognizes PPPD in the same way there is a quick and simple test for say, the flu[41]. Rather, diagnosis of PPPD requires a set of specific criteria – which we will outline shortly – to be met[21]. Therefore, identification of PPPD in a patient requires a series of events that collectively allows the practitioner to arrive at a final diagnosis of PPPD.

Medical history

One of the most valuable bits of information is the patient's medical history[41]. Patients who have reached the point at which they seek medical attention for PPPD have been described as being at their 'wits end', an indication of just how involved but also how misunderstood the condition of PPPD can be[21]. In a best-case scenario of PPPD, patients will report a mild type of dizziness that is often hard to describe[41]. The dizziness is worsened when in an upright position, when moving such as walking or if in a car, and in environments in which there is a lot of visual stimulation, such as a movie theater, driving on a road full of shadows, or perhaps when walking on carpet with a unique pattern. Additional patient history can help separate out a likelihood of other vestibular events. For example, if patients feel dizziness or vertigo when looking up at the ceiling or perhaps when rolling over in bed, it is expected that they would be suffering from BPPV as compared to PPPD. Because of the numerous other conditions that mimic PPPD, patients must be sure to provide a detailed medical history when discussing their symptoms with their medical provider. For patients suspected of having PPPD, it is expected that they will initially undergo the standard vestibular workup. This can include aspects that test for balance such as videonystagmography, positional tests, caloric testing of the ear, or head impulse tests, among others[16]. Positional tests can include something as simple as monitoring the degree of body sway that occurs when standing, as patients with PPPD will show increased sway in addition to likely arm movement to compensate for the swaying[21]. Balance can be checked quickly with a simple procedure such as the Romberg test which requires that the patient stand stationary with his or her eyes closed[54]. If a patient sways excessively back and forth, or if they fall to one side, it can be indicative of a vestibular issue or an inability to receive and process information about one's body position[55], both of which could fall under PPPD.

Similarly, gait analysis can be used to assess for issues within a patient's central nervous system which may reveal problems in the brain's ability to process vestibular signals. For example, a *walking Romberg* test requires only that a patient walk normally for five meters with their eyes closed[54]. If there is any swaying, noted instability, or an inability to complete the distance without opening their eyes, it can suggest a complication with balance processing[56]. When dealing with PPPD, even simple observation of an individual's gait can reveal a degree of hesitation when walking, much like what might be observed when someone is attempting to walk on ice[21].

In addition to physical tests, surveys can be used to evaluate the degree of disability that a patient experiences[16]. Examples of these surveys can include the Vestibular Rehabilitation Benefit Questionnaire, the Dizziness Handicap Inventory, and the Nijmegen Questionnaire[16]. And in a bit of good news for PPPD patients, a questionnaire has recently been developed that has been shown to be highly reliable and valid for assessing the severity of PPPD[39].

Patients suspected to have PPPD will likely have normal diagnostic test results[16]. Surveys, on the other hand, may show significant impact of the disease on their daily life. Imaging studies such as magnetic resonance (i.e. "MRI") will also likely be normal in patients with PPPD[16], unless some other condition (e.g. acoustic neuroma) is contributing to their symptoms. However, the emerging field of *posturography* has shown that PPPD patients often score worse at maintaining postural control than patients who previously had a vestibular condition but were able to make a full recovery[57].

Because of the potential for anxiety or other psychological contributions to PPPD, some researchers recommend a psychological screening as part of the overall PPPD evaluation[16]. This screening can be done using specific surveys such as the Health Anxiety Inventory which is designed to reveal aspects that are relevant to PPPD.

Diagnostic Criteria

For a patient to be diagnosed with PPPD they must meet all five of the criteria used to identify PPPD. Those criteria, as written by the committee for the Classification of Vestibular Disorders of the Barany Society are as follows[35]:

A. **One or more symptoms of dizziness, unsteadiness, or non-spinning vertigo are present on most days for 3 months or more.**
1. Symptoms last for prolonged (hours-long) periods of time, but may wax and wane in severity.
2. Symptoms need not be present continuously throughout the entire day.

B. **Persistent symptoms occur without specific provocation, but are exacerbated by three factors:**
1. Upright posture
2. Active or passive motion without regard to direction or position
3. Exposure to moving visual stimuli or complex visual patterns

C. **The disorder is precipitated by conditions that cause vertigo, unsteadiness, dizziness, or problems with balance including acute, episodic, or chronic vestibular syndromes, other**

neurologic or medical illnesses, or psychological distress

1. When the precipitant is an acute or episodic condition, symptoms settle into the pattern of criterion "A" as the precipitant resolves, but they may occur intermittently at first, and then consolidate into a persistent course.

2. When the precipitant is a chronic syndrome, symptoms may develop slowly at first and worsen gradually

D. Symptoms cause significant distress or functional impairment

E. Symptoms are not better accounted for by another disease or disorder

As noted, for a patient to be diagnosed with PPPD he or she must meet all of the criteria listed[35]. This does not mean that a patient will not have some sort of variance in their degree of symptoms. For example, a patient does not have to say that he or she specifically experiences 'dizziness' to be diagnosed with PPPD. They may claim to experience lightheadedness, cloudiness, or even a type of 'fullness' that can be grouped in with dizziness[35]. Similarly, a patient does not have to claim specifically that they have vertigo. Rather, they may instead report a swaying motion, rocking, or any other descriptions of perceived motion[35].

In addition to the diagnostic criteria listed earlier, researchers have also outlined a summary of PPPD specific to its clinical-based characteristics[16]. These include the following:

- Persistent sensations of unsteadiness and/or non-vertiginous dizziness lasting 3 or more months
- Symptoms present on more days than not (at least 15 days of the last 30)
- Symptoms worsen with an upright posture, head or body motion, or exposure to complex or motion-rich environments
- Symptoms lessen or are absent in a reclined or resting posture
- Absence of currently active medical or neurological conditions, or use of any medication, both of which may cause dizziness
- Results from radiographic imaging exclude significant anatomical lesions
- Findings from balance function tests are within normal limits, reveal deficits not believed to be currently active, or cannot fully explain all of the patient's symptoms

We also discussed in an earlier chapter that some patients may experience brief periods in which their symptoms are minimally present. This is rare[35], and should not be taken as an improvement in the patient's PPPD. Some patients have an on-again, off-again phase of symptoms early in the course of PPPD, while others have a relatively slow but continual onset of symptoms[35]. Either scenario can still qualify as having a true case of PPPD.

In diagnosing PPPD, it is also important to recognize when a patient's symptoms are NOT indicative of PPPD. Such situations are largely based upon the patient's medical history as well as their diagnostic test results. For example, if they do not have a positive result for physician-driven tests such as a head-thrust test or balance testing, PPPD is a more likely diagnosis[35]. But if there is vertigo in response to motion or other findings that are more consistent with a different vestibular condition, PPPD will likely be ruled out[35]. Such a situation may arise if a patient claims that they have sudden dizziness when standing, but the dizziness only occurs when they look up at the ceiling. Even though the fact that an upright posture would suggest PPPD, the requirement that the patient must be looking at the ceiling for the dizziness to occur might be more relevant of BPPV than PPPD.

Such a situation highlights the fact that many vestibular conditions have symptoms that closely mimic each other. This can make an accurate diagnosis difficult to ascertain, and patients should be aware that it may take a significant amount of testing in order to clearly identify a particular diagnosis. In addition, as PPPD is triggered by an initial vestibular event (e.g. vestibular neuritis), it is important to determine whether a patient's current symptoms are due to lingering effects of that initial condition or whether the symptoms are in fact due to the presence of PPPD. Proper treatment is dependent upon an accurate diagnosis, so it is vital that your medical provider has all the information necessary to make the correct diagnosis.

Conclusion

Diagnosis of PPPD is dependent upon a specific set of diagnostic criteria. Patients who are experiencing dizziness and/or vertigo could be suffering from a variety of vestibular conditions, and medical professionals often have to apply a battery of tests in order to determine whether a patient is indeed suffering from PPPD or any of a number of similar medical conditions. Still, once the proper diagnosis has been determined, treatment can be applied in order to attempt to improve the patient's condition. In the next chapter we will look at several of the treatment options that are available for PPPD patients. In consultation with a patient's medical provider, it is anticipated that a diagnosis of PPPD can allow for a personalized treatment plan to counteract the negative effects of this disease.

Chapter 5 – Treatment of PPPD

THE PATHWAY TO A CURE for any disease involves steps that include recognition of symptoms, a proper diagnosis, and finally an individualized treatment plan. For many vestibular disorders like PPPD, the lack of understanding of a mechanism for the disease makes treatment somewhat difficult in that there is not a clear outline of what structures or phenomenon is causing the condition. Therefore, treatment often starts out as a trial-and-error process in which the patient records his or her successes along with those events that tend to worsen their condition. Given the relative newness of PPPD, treatment has yet to be clearly outlined. However, as we progress with understanding this disease we will also continue to build a framework of the most successful treatments that can in turn be refined to improve future treatment plans for PPPD patients.

As stated throughout this book, PPPD is not a 'structural' condition in that it is not directly tied to one particular body organ in the same way that complications from a fracture can be tied to a broken bone.

Consequently, patients may have difficulty in understanding just what the source of their symptoms actually is. *Am I having a stroke? Will I ever be normal again? What happens if I fall and get injured?* Those are all potential questions that a patient may be constantly asking themselves. Therefore, one of the first treatment steps is to ensure that your medical provider thoroughly informs you of the condition[58]. Doing so can help ensure that you learn that it is in fact *not* "all in your head", or that you "just need to relax more".

Vestibular Rehabilitation

Vestibular rehabilitation is a type of therapy that involves working to improve a patient's remaining balance function, or in some cases help an undamaged inner ear compensate for the opposite one that has been compromised. Vestibular exercises can be beneficial for patients of dizziness[59]. With PPPD, vestibular rehabilitation aims to 'calm down' a seemingly hyperactive vestibular system[60]. This is done through the use of habituation exercises as well as relaxation techniques[60]. However, it must be noted that treatment which incorporates vestibular rehabilitation has the potential to aggravate PPPD symptoms, thereby negating any vestibular rehabilitation benefit[20]. This is not to say that vestibular rehabilitation should not be incorporated into a PPPD patient's treatment plan, but rather that patients and medical providers should recognize that the

76

potential for aggravation of a patient's PPPD symptoms could occur.

Examples of physical-oriented vestibular rehabilitation can include aspects such as a walking program, where the goal is to maintain a brisk walk for 30 minutes. Additionally, patients may be recommended to perform exercises that are capable of inducing dizziness within a very controlled situation[58]. Separately, visual-based therapies can involve motion screens or virtual reality in order to help desensitize patients to motion[58].

Due to the psychological aspect that PPPD often involves, it may be necessary to also incorporate anxiety-specific treatments along with any other psychological aspects[20]. For example, PPPD patients might be told that it is acceptable to maintain an awareness of their dizziness (as PPPD patients often do), but to avoid allowing it to cause anxiety[58]. Additional efforts should focus on the importance of getting a good night's sleep, engaging in adequate physical activity, and maintaining a healthy diet[20].

Because PPPD is such a new medical condition, there is not a lot of information specific to the benefits of vestibular rehabilitation on PPPD. Rather, most information is taken from some of the related conditions such as chronic subjective dizziness. For example, over half of patients with chronic subjective dizziness reported that vestibular rehabilitation either reduced or eliminated their symptoms[61]. Given the known benefits of vestibular rehabilitation on dizziness disorders that are similar to

PPPD, it should be expected that as more PPPD patients are identified, the specific benefits of vestibular rehabilitation in this population will be identified through directed research.

Cognitive behavior therapy

The link between a physical and psychological component with PPPD makes cognitive behavior therapy a viable treatment option for patients. The aim of CBT is to reduce the effects of a particular psychological condition (e.g. anxiety) through repeated exposure. This occurs through directed therapy such as thorough patient education about the condition, identification of triggers and the subsequent patient response (e.g. anxiety, avoidance of public places, etc.), and desensitization exercises to suspected triggers as well as the patient responses[62]. A main theory behind CBT is that as the individual is exposed to anxiety-related situations repeatedly in a controlled setting, he or she begins to experience less anxiety. Even a brief CBT intervention by a trained psychologist can have the effect of reducing dizziness in patients[62]. Furthermore, CBT has been shown to positively influence dizziness. Among patients who were exposed to dizziness-provoking situations but encouraged *not* to dwell on having a dizziness-related condition, almost one-fourth later ended up symptom-free while half reported considerable improvement[63].

CBT has been shown to be effective at treating the conditions associated with PPPD[62]. For example, patients with phobic postural vertigo who purposely caused at least two dizzying events per day and then received CBT in conjunction with vestibular rehabilitation reported greater reduction in anxiety and depression than patients who received the vestibular rehabilitation only[64]. However, the researchers pointed out that the improvements seen were not still present one year later during follow-up[65]. This is not necessarily a negative finding of CBT, though, as it simply means that more studies are needed to look directly at the effects of CBT in patients who have been specifically diagnosed with PPPD.

Medication

Certain prescription medications have been used to help reduce the symptoms of dizziness. Selective serotonin reuptake inhibitors (SSRI) along with serotonin-norepinephrine reuptake inhibitors (SNRI)) are drugs that are commonly prescribed in patients who report chronic dizziness[40] and have been shown to be effective at reducing the symptoms that occur with PPPD[66]. Unfortunately, the side effects of this class of medication as well as a perceived lack of positive effects can drive patients to stop use of these drugs[58]. Still, up to two-thirds of patients report beneficial effects, indicating that the drugs have the potential to be a positive therapy for PPPD patients[58]. In fact, the success of these drugs has led them to be the most popular treatment for PPPD[67]. Interestingly, the addition of the SSRI drug sertraline in conjunction with CBT was found to be effective in treating PPPD, and the combined therapy even required a lower dose of the sertraline drug[67].

It has also been noted that drugs which suppress the vestibular system, such as medications that are taken for nausea or car-sickness (e.g. antihistamines, benzodiazepenes, and others) are not generally recommended as a therapy for patients with symptoms such as PPPD as they can negatively impact a patient's rehabilitation[58, 68].

Nerve stimulation

The use of therapeutic electrical stimulation is a relatively new treatment option for PPPD patients. For example, vagus nerve stimulation has been shown to be effective at reducing the effects of depression[69] in addition to lessening the severity of certain headaches[70]. When the vagus nerve was stimulated in PPPD patients, depression scores improved along with an improvement in quality of life[71]. Perhaps more importantly, these same patients reported a decrease in the severity of their dizziness attacks as well as a diminished amount of postural sway.

Similarly, when electrical stimulation was applied in 30 minute bouts over five days to the prefrontal cortex of the brain of PPPD patients, those patients reported a reduction in dizziness on the days that they received the electrical stimulation treatment[72]. Unfortunately, the days following the treatments did not maintain the reduction in dizziness, but even the brief improvement in dizziness suggest that future research could help reveal how electrical stimulation may be a potential target for helping improve not only quality of life but also reducing the symptoms of PPPD.

Conclusion

The treatment of PPPD is one of the newest areas of vestibular rehabilitation. As such, there is not a wealth of data or existing research to base PPPD treatment protocols on. Therefore, medicine is still in a trial-and-error phase of treatment for PPPD, whereby treatments are largely based either on successes from treating similar vestibular conditions (e.g. PPV, depression, etc.) or are largely theoretical-based. Currently, successful treatments target the psychological side of PPPD as well as re-educating the vestibular system. As these and other treatments become more focused and the available research continues to broaden, it should follow that more effective treatments will soon become available to PPPD patients.

Chapter 6 – My story

IN THE INTEREST of full disclosure, it's necessary for me to point out that despite writing this book, I have never been officially diagnosed with PPPD. My own vestibular conditions began long before the official recognition of PPPD and while the effects of my disorders span the range of mildly annoying to extremely debilitating, they have largely been under control for almost the past 10 years. Still, I randomly have bouts of anxiety or a sudden imbalance that not only reminds me that my vestibular issues still lurk, but also make me question whether I exhibit the characteristic symptoms of PPPD or one of its similar conditions. In this chapter, I'll detail some of the more significant balance and instability issues I've experienced during my time dealing with vestibular disorders.

In the early 2000s I was diagnosed with and successfully treated for BPPV. While treatment of BPPV now requires just a quick and simple Epley maneuver that can be done at home, the fact that I was afflicted with during its early days of discovery meant that I was relegated to 48 hours of wearing a soft neck brace and not allowing my head or torso to waver from a vertical position. But I made it through and was left symptom-free from vestibular issues until a few years later when I noticed tinnitus in my right ear that eventually moved to my left. In 2011 I was diagnosed with Ménière's disease after about 3 years of relevant symptoms that included several drop attacks as well as severe anxiety and dizziness. In between all of this, I went through a period during which I had a continual headache of some degree for over a year, which when combined with certain vestibular symptoms that I experienced at the time led some to believe that I was also suffering from some degree of vestibular migraine. But again, all of these – with the exception of the tinnitus that is now more prominent in my left ear – are largely under control. The vast majority of symptoms subsided after I switched to a very-low-sodium diet as required for my Ménière's disease. The full details of each of the conditions I experienced are documented in my other vestibular books.

Despite being significantly better now than when I was experiencing each of my conditions, I am certainly not saying that I don't still experience random vestibular symptoms. I still get occasional reminders that my own dizziness-related conditions have not been cured but rather are lurking just under the surface. Despite no official diagnosis, many of the symptoms that I either have had or still do experience are eerily similar to those symptoms reported by PPPD patients. Therefore, I'll next outline a few of those PPPD-associated symptoms to give you my own perspective.

Uneven walking surfaces

Walking on a perfectly flat surface such as a building floor was never an issue for me. The problem was that if the surface had any type of tilt or slope to it that I wasn't aware of, it quickly became *very* problematic. A sudden tingling-type jolt up my back followed soon after by a racing heartbeat, along with my exhibiting a minor type of "parachute reflex" that babies display as they shoot their arms out to break a fall. Clearly evident slopes were not an issue, as I could prepare to adjust my body position or gait appropriately. Rather, it was the very small perturbations on a walking surface that set me off, as the change registered within my input sensors (likely my feet) but was not calmly 'accepted' by my brain. Such a situation occurred most often on outdoor sidewalks that had a small, almost undetectable change in slope. A few times I even had to stop walking to adjust myself visually to the alteration in the surface. Over time I began to adjust to and recognize where the unexpected changes in the walking surface were at, which in turn helped reduce the frequency of these events.

It wasn't just the walking surface itself that could cause problems but also any unexpected change to my gait. For example, there were many times in which I had a balance issue while on a flat surface but was pushed slightly sideways by a gust of wind. Rather than simply accepting the adjustment to my walking pattern and continuing on, I had to instead put forth a significant amount of mental processing, even at times stopping to 'reset' my sensors. Strangely, I don't recall ever having fallen due to any of these events, so there seemed to be no need to be extremely anxious about such situations. Still, the amount of anxiety that even a miniscule but unexpected change could cause was shocking to me, to the point that it further contributed to my constantly thinking about my vestibular status.

Long Hallways

When I was symptomatic, I worked in a research hospital that had a very simple rectangular floorplan design. This meant that to get around a particular floor you would walk a path along two very long hallways and two rather short hallways. The long hallways were always problematic for me – so much that I would intentionally walk next to one of the walls so that I would have the ability to brace myself if needed. There was nothing unique about the hallway – just a white tile floor with white painted walls intermixed with door frames, medical posters, or display cases. But for some reason, looking down the length of those hallways would affect me in ways that none others seemed to in that it would bring on instant unsteadiness. Even knowing that I would need to walk out in the hallway at some point in the near future would trigger a degree of low-level anxiety for me. If I was in charge of when I would need to be in the hallway, it was a relatively mild case that slowly progressed as the point at which I needed to make the trip approached. Much worse was when a co-worker or my boss would give me a directive that required me to head out into the hallway with no warning. That would start my heart racing, and always made the trip itself much worse than it should have been. Truth be told, nothing ever *actually* happened; rather, it just felt constantly like something was *about* to happen when walking in the halls – an 'aura' of sorts that made it seem like at any second I was about to have a very strong vestibular attack.

Trying to explain what the feeling was like when actually in the hallway is quite difficult, much like any time when trying to explain any psychological problem. Obviously there is a strong degree of nervousness mixed in with a bit of fear that something is about to happen. For me, it felt as though the hallway was 'closing in' on me, similar to that movie effect known as the "dolly zoom", often used in scenes of fear or terror (and ironically first used in an Alfred Hitchcock film called *Vertigo*!). The effect also triggered some strange pressure feeling in my face, an odd but very present sensation that I grew to despise. Nevertheless, upon entering those long hallways, my thoughts were instantly directed 100% towards my vestibular condition – to the point that it was difficult to even focus on a conversation, or at least to the point that I was afraid that any conversation I engaged in would reveal that I was in a bit of a panic at the moment.

Interestingly, since having gone on a low-sodium diet for my Ménière's, this strange effect in the hallway disappeared and has remained suppressed for many years.

Stairwells

Alongside difficulty with long hallways was the problem of stairwells. One run of straight stairs was never an issue – it was the winding shaft of stairs located at the end of a hallway that caused me difficulty. The problem for me was quite pronounced when going *down* the stairs – something about looking down while turning repetitively caused me quite a bit of anxiety and lingering dizziness. Therefore, I adopted a unique and probably odd-looking technique in that I would turn my body separately from my head. When going down stairs and reaching a particular stairwell landing I would turn my body to keep going down more stairs, but turning of my head back to the neutral (i.e. face-forward) position would occur a second or two later. This seemed to reduce the eventual dizziness and also served to reduce my anxiety. I even adopted this disjointed strategy during times when I had to navigate my way across a crowded room that required me to twist and turn to avoid obstacles, similar to what might be required to get from one end of a classroom to another through a group of unevenly-spaced desks. Even today, I am cognizant of the potential effects of going down a circular stairwell, but the effects are not as prominent now as when I was having my associated vestibular disorders.

Driving

One of my longest-lasting symptoms has been an intermittent issue that I still experience when driving, even after having switched to a low-sodium diet. Initially, when my symptoms first started, wide roads such as three- and four-lane freeways were problematic. City streets, particularly those in which I didn't get much over 45 miles per hour, were not much of an issue while interstates through big cities – with seemingly endless overpasses and at times 4 to 5 lanes of traffic – induced anxiety that made driving a difficult task. It wasn't a fear of driving that caused the problem – rather it was the sensation induced by the wide field of vision on those four-lane highways. Even worse were the overpasses, as I would have to grip the steering wheel to further 'confirm' that I was indeed sitting in a car and not falling backwards as I drove up the overpass.

As my symptoms worsened over time, I noticed a particular problem when driving on what I consider "bouncy" roads. These were roads, usually at a higher speed, which caused my car to bounce up and down forcefully. Rough roads, such as those where the concrete was cracked or potholes existed, were not a problem. Rather, it was the sudden and powerful up-and-down bouncing in my seat that could lead to minor and repetitive anxiety attacks. This effect still occurs even today, though to a much lower degree than back when I was experiencing all of my vestibular symptoms.

Another big problem that remains is continued anxiety on high overpasses. For most of my life I had no problem with heights, whether that be from climbing, driving over bridges, or just being in a tall building. But as my own vestibular conditions evolved, I noticed that bridges and then overpasses began to cause me anxiety, first at a very minor level before getting to the point where I would do whatever I could to avoid driving over them. On multiple instances I found myself on an overpass with concrete barriers on the side. This served to block my view of any land, leaving me only the view of the sky against the road in front of my vehicle. And if there was a curve in the overpass or bridge, the panic was heightened even more as my body would feel a tilt that set off warning signals about my body position relevant to what my visual input was registering – mainly that I was falling backwards.

I had several panic attacks occur in this situation before I was able to understand the underlying link to my vestibular disorders. It got to the point that even going up a hill could be problematic, such that if I saw the sky touching the road up in front of me it would trigger issues with my equilibrium, especially if I felt myself being pushed back into my seat when going up the hill. Clouds would help provide some perspective for my brain to lock onto, but a clear blue sky when going up an overpass was especially nerve-wracking. As I reached the top of the overpass and started heading downward, though, the view of the surrounding ground seemed to make everything fall back to normal again. Still today I get a bit apprehensive when approaching overpasses, though it's not nearly as bad as when I was suffering the effects of what I was told was a Ménière's diagnosis.

Chapter 7 – Predecessors of PPPD

PPPD HAS ONLY GAINED a foothold in the medical community over the past decade or so. During this time, several medical conditions were grouped together into what we now know as PPPD. Prior to combining these conditions into PPPD, they existed independently, albeit with several overlapping symptoms between each that often made it difficult to separate one from another. Because they are independent conditions, each comes with its own specific symptoms, triggers, and complications. Therefore, in this chapter we'll take a look at some of these medical conditions that eventually became known as PPPD and outline the symptoms associated with each. Whereas the information that the medical community has gathered about each condition over the years has served to provide us the collective information that we now know about PPPD, I think it's important that we outline each condition individually to better understand how our knowledge of PPPD has evolved.

Visual Vertigo

A certain proportion of dizzy patients report that their symptoms increase when in a very 'busy' visual environment[73], a condition known as *visual vertigo* (VV). Visual vertigo is a long-standing condition in which a chronic dizziness or balance scenario has led to a greater dependence on visual input of one's environment[74]. Examples of environments that can be problematic for VV sufferers include driving or when walking in supermarket aisles, and patients generally are not comfortable with actively moving surroundings such as crowds or disco lights[73]. In fact, most patients of VV actually have more than one specific trigger[30], and VV patients often report an increase in their symptoms when placed in an environment that is heavy with visual activity[30].

It has been suspected that visual vertigo results from a vestibular disorder that occurs in conjunction with a panic or anxiety disorder[75]. Specifically, patients tend to have conflicting input between their visual and perceptual (e.g. head motion, foot sensors) receptors, in turn relying more on visual input to make movement decisions[76].

Phobic Postural Vertigo

Phobic postural vertigo (PPV) has been identified as one of the most common disorders that is presented at ear clinics[34]. Unfortunately, it is not always recognized when occurring in a patient[34], which may explain its widely reported prevalence range among dizziness clinic patients of anywhere from 2.5% of diagnoses[77] to 23%[78]. As a medical condition, PPV has several symptoms and characteristics[34]. These include PPV often starting after an initial inner-ear disorder such as vestibular neuritis, after which patients complain of dizziness and unsteadiness that is not evident to others and does not dissipate. This initial event is followed by intense attacks related to a fear of falling, as well as attacks that occur in specific areas such as driving over a bridge or in a crowded restaurant. Symptoms seem to subside during activity such as exercise but can reappear when resting, and it has been noted that a slight amount of alcohol seems to alleviate symptoms for some patients. Furthermore, like many of the dizziness conditions, there tends to be a bit of psychiatric personality issues such as obsessive-compulsive disorder in conjunction with the disease.

Most vestibular-based testing is normal in patients with PPV[34]. This in turn is somewhat of a problem for diagnosis, as given the fact that vestibular tests are typically negative with PPV, accepting that there is indeed a vestibular-based issue can be problematic[34]. Still, patients with PPV have been shown to have a greater degree of postural sway during standing activities[79], and this imbalance tends to increase when PPV patients are exposed to moving scenes[34]. PPV patients have also been shown to exhibit an increased level of stiffened postural muscles[80].

Because there is a psychological aspect of PPV in conjunction with often-negative vestibular tests, receiving a PPV diagnosis often takes years and involves multiple specialists. One study found an average of 3 years between the initiation of symptoms and a final diagnosis[81], certainly problematic for a patient suffering the effects of a vestibular condition such as PPV. Furthering the frustration is that during the time it takes to obtain a correct diagnosis, patients are often misdiagnosed with other conditions such as recurrent *vertebrobasilar ischemia* or *cervicogenic vertigo*[82], followed by unsuccessful treatment that leads the patient to seek additional medical care.

The underlying issue that triggers the effects of PPV is not known. At best, it is theorized that there is some sort of disconnect in PPV patients that does not correlate the act of voluntarily moving with the feedback received from that movement[28]. Couple that characteristic with a likely anxiety issue that calls for constant checking and re-checking of one's balance, and PPV can be the result.

Chronic subjective dizziness

One of the predecessors of PPPD has only been around for about the last couple of decades. *Chronic subjective dizziness*, or "CSD", was built off of the information available for PPV. Much like PPV, CSD often exists quite some time before diagnosis. One study reported that patients took over four years to get seen by a specialist[33], suspected to be due to the lack of understanding of PPV even by vestibular specialists. And much like PPPD, diagnosis of CSD requires several criteria to be met[33] including persistent dizziness, light-headedness, or imbalance on most days for the past 3 months or more, constant awareness of one's own movement, and an increase in symptoms when the patient is in visually-stimulating environments such as a busy market or when using a computer. However, as a vestibular condition CSD can also exist in conjunction with other vestibular disorders[40], making it particularly problematic to diagnose if other conditions also exist.

While CSD is in fact quite similar to PPV, there are also important differences[34]. For example, CSD focuses more on the chronic unsteadiness and dizziness that a patient experiences, whereas PPV outlines specific attacks that can occur. Furthermore, CSD is more directed toward motion-induced triggers than PPV. And CSD has more emphasis on the psychological component of the disease whereas PPV is focused more on postural-based aspects of the disease.

Conclusion

While each of the three diseases discussed in this chapter have been identified as independent conditions, they are now treated collectively as PPPD. While PPPD itself is quite new as a medical condition, the research accumulated through studying visual vertigo, phobic postural vertigo, and chronic subjective dizziness have provided a foundation of research that can now be built on as researchers and medical professionals turn their attention towards PPPD itself. In doing so, and as more characteristics of PPPD patients are revealed, it should be expected that the true underlying cause of PPPD will be revealed. And, once a cause has been outlined, treatments and therapies can be designed that focus on the specific tissue or pathology responsible for triggering the effects of PPPD.

Chapter 8 – Patient Experiences

AS A PATIENT OF PPPD, you probably have your own unique set of symptoms that you deal with in your own life. In this chapter, I have collected a variety of patient-documented experiences that outline what a day is like with PPPD from their own individual viewpoint. Given the wide variety of experiences that different patients have after being diagnosed with PPPD, I thought it would be beneficial for you to see what other patients experience with this disease on a daily basis. The purpose of these narratives are not to frighten you or give you a negative outlook of what life will be like with PPPD. Rather, they are included here with the intent of helping you understand that your own difficulties with PPPD are shared by many others. Therefore, read this chapter with caution as some perspectives make PPPD seem like quite a debilitating disease, which it may or may not be for you specifically.

I first had some dizziness at work, then again 1 week later in a big market, and again a few days later while waiting at the eye doctor. I was brought to urgent care who then told me to go to vestibular physiotherapy for inner-ear crystal repositioning. I spent the next two months on the sofa. I could not walk. At the hospital they provided several treatments for BPPV, tinnitus, migraine, neck pain, blocked ears, intracranial pressure, but nothing worked. Diamox helped me. It has been 9 months since diagnosis that I have gone to vestibular physiotherapy, and it is getting better very slowly. Light, movement, and sound are my real enemies. The only place here I feel well is out in nature without any visual pollution. I feel optimistic but I am also wondering what will happen with my job. And I have no social life at the moment, as that is impossible for me.

Isolating. Debilitating. Terrifying. These are just a few of the words that come to mind when I think of my life right now. And one of the most frustrating aspects of my experience is the fact that my illnesses – the beasts that have altered every aspect of my being – are invisible. On the outside, I look just like everyone else. But on the inside, I have two chronic illnesses that are wreaking havoc on my entire body. Yes, most people will understand on a logical level that I have PPPD and chronic migraines and that they impact my daily life. But they don't feel what I feel: the dizziness and the pain. It's difficult for some people to understand, to believe even, that when I get out of an elevator I feel as if a minor earthquake is happening. The ground shakes beneath my feet and I feel as if I am swaying from side to side. And when I feel the need to walk it is always close to a wall and without looking down, because my vision is going blurry and the stripes on the carpet are too much to take in at the moment. I sometimes feel as if I'm being judged. It's also difficult for some people to understand that simple, everyday tasks like cooking, cleaning, and doing laundry are almost impossible for me to do anymore without me feeling as if I'm swaying and as if my head just isn't on quite right. It's difficult for people who don't have PPPD to understand these sensations and feelings because they haven't experienced them themselves: They haven't experienced how grabbing an onion from the fridge, and then the cutting board from the other side of the kitchen, and then the knife from beside the sink – and how all of the associated motions that go along with this seemingly simple task – can make it feel as if the room is spinning and can make my head pain spike, and all in under a minute or two. They haven't experienced how getting up from the couch too fast and walking 10 feet to the bathroom too quickly before realizing it can make me incredibly dizzy and set my day back. They haven't experienced how the tiny act of moving my head from one side of the pillow to the other can send intense bursts of pain through my head, enough to make it so I can't fall asleep again for over an hour. They just haven't experienced life with PPPD and chronic migraines. I guess what it really comes down to is this: Everything is a trigger it seems – movement, sounds, light, strong smells. So, I've created a bubble around myself. My world has become incredibly small, and the four walls I live in have become an isolation chamber of sorts. Living with the dizziness and the pain associated with my PPPD and chronic migraines is one thing. But honestly, for me, the isolation – the fact that my reality is shrinking and shrinking because of my illnesses – is the most debilitating part. And, the fact that I still look like the old me on the outside and some people still expect me to be that old version of myself, when, in actuality, I really don't know who I am anymore: That fact terrifies me. So, there you have it. PPPD hasn't just made me dizzy. It hasn't just increased my pain. PPPD has changed everything.

PPPD is like my mood – sometimes you feel like it's a good day with mild feelings of being spaced-out or dizzy or fatigued. But those days are just mild – it doesn't take up a huge part in your conscious mind. On bad days, when you don't sleep or eat well, or when you feel stressed, you feel you are highly irritated, just like that feeling when you don't sleep - but at a higher level. Then you combine that feeling with the anxiety about why you feel this way, which distorts your feelings more and creates even more depression.

Chapter 9 - Related Conditions

VESTIBULAR-RELATED SYMPTOMS come in many shapes and sizes and are all capable of causing significant disability for the patient. The symptoms associated with PPPD often resemble those found with other inner-ear conditions, and as such it is of interest to note the *differences* that can exist between the many vestibular conditions which can cause symptoms such as unsteadiness, tinnitus, or hearing loss. Therefore, this chapter is designed to outline some of the more common medical conditions that can mimic the signs and symptoms associated with PPPD. In doing so, it not only highlights the similarities with PPPD but also outlines some key differences that can help medical professionals isolate PPPD as a potential culprit behind a patient's symptoms.

Ménière's disease

Ménière's disease is an illness thought to result from problems with the fluid regulation system of the inner ear. Ménière's patients typically experience an ongoing degree of unsteadiness and ear pressure or fullness intermixed with bouts of acute vertigo, nausea, and vomiting that can last several hours or more. Due in large part to the complexity and sensitivity of the vestibular system, Ménière's remains a complicated disease. While the acute vertigo attacks of Ménière's can be extremely debilitating, those attacks can be followed by months or years of almost no symptoms.

Several theorized causes of Ménière's have been proposed, including body water regulation issues, endolymph reabsorption anomalies, vascular abnormalities, and autoimmune factors. Of these possible causes, fluid regulation in the middle ear is considered to be one of the main triggers of Ménière's[83]. For example, water channels, which regulate the transport of water across membranes, have been implicated as a possible main cause of Ménière's[84]. This theory results from the idea that unexpected reductions or increases in the number of water channels can influence the balance of fluid on each side of a membrane, and any alteration in fluid balance can have negative consequences in the equilibrium system of the ear.

Similarly, some researchers suggest that Ménière's patients have a diminished capacity to regulate fluid within their inner ear[85]. Consequently, fluctuations in the inner ear fluid are not well tolerated in Ménière's patients. This is thought to lead to fluid imbalances that contribute to many of the symptoms encountered by Ménière's patients. Electrolytes such as sodium that are known to play a role in the body's fluid regulation are commonly restricted in Ménière's patients in order to reduce potential fluctuations within the middle ear.

Other theorized causes of Ménière's disease include autoimmune disorders[86], the herpes virus[87], cervical (i.e. neck) disorders[88] and stress[89]. Whereas no definitive cause of Ménière's has been discovered, it is vital that research continue to investigate these and all logical possibilities to determine the potential link and/or similarities between Ménière's and PPPD. At present there remains no cure for Ménière's, though symptoms can often be controlled through the aforementioned sodium restriction, medication, intratympanic steroid injection, and if necessary, surgical procedures on the middle ear.

Benign positional paroxysmal vertigo

As we have discussed, one of the most common vertigo conditions seen in primary care is benign positional paroxysmal vertigo (BPPV)[90]. Despite the long name, each word plays a role in describing what occurs with the disease. Most patients with this relatively harmless (benign) condition describe sudden (i.e. paroxysmal) bouts of vertigo that occur with certain positional-dependent head positions.

The mechanism involved in BPPV is thought to be due to the presence of loose crystals (i.e. otoliths) within the semicircular canals of the ear. As otoliths are not normally present within the semicircular canals, certain head movements cause the loose otoliths to contact the delicate hair cells of the semicircular canals, causing them to trigger and falsely indicate body motion when the head is in particular positions. For example, patients with BPPV often report short bouts of vertigo when looking upwards or rolling over in bed[91]. Furthermore, nausea and vomiting can occur with more severe cases such as *intractable BPPV*.

Diagnosis of BPPV typically involves a thorough medical history and evaluation along with manipulating the head in an attempt to reproduce the symptoms. Most commonly, the Dix-Hallpike maneuver is used to attempt to reproduce the symptoms of BPPV. For this procedure, the patient is seated on a table and their head position is manipulated while the patient is put through a series of specific body positions. Because the otoliths will typically induce nystagmus along with vertigo, the patient's eyes are observed for nystagmus along with any patient-reported vertigo. Results of the Dix-Hallpike test are relatively reliable, being able to correctly identify patients with BPPV 83% of the time while correctly excluding patients without BPPV 52% of the time[90].

For those patients testing positive for BPPV, vestibular rehabilitation as well as canalith repositioning (e.g. Epley maneuver) are relatively successful. Vestibular rehabilitation typically consists of a series of head and/or body motions which may involve fixation of the eye on a single point. Pharmaceutical treatments are not recommended for use in the treatment of BPPV as research has shown no benefit[92]. It is also possible that BBPV symptoms return.

Vestibular migraine

Vestibular migraines are among the more common vestibular disorders, affecting up to 1% of the population[93, 94] and up to 11% of patients seeking treatment in dizziness-related clinics[95]. Vestibular migraines are also relatively common in children, having been reported to occur in nearly 3% of children aged 6-12 years of age[96]. Like Ménière's disease, vestibular migraine has no universally accepted definition, which can in turn limit recognition of vestibular migraines in affected patients. Only recently were the diagnostic criteria established which include the following[95].

1. Vestibular migraine

A. At least 5 episodes with vestibular symptoms of moderate or severe intensity, lasting 5 minutes to 72 hours

B. Current or previous history of migraine with or without aura according to the International Classification of Headache Disorders (ICHD)

C. One or more migraine features with at least 50% of the vestibular episodes:

− headache with at least two of the following characteristics: one sided location, pulsating quality, moderate or severe pain intensity, aggravation by routine physical activity

− photophobia and phonophobia

− visual aura

D. Not better accounted for by another vestibular or ICHD diagnosis

    2. Probable vestibular migraine

    A. At least 5 episodes with vestibular symptoms of moderate or severe intensity, lasting 5 min to 72 hours

    B. Only one of the criteria B and C for vestibular migraine is fulfilled (migraine history or migraine features during the episode)

    C. Not better accounted for by another vestibular or ICHD diagnosis

The predominant symptoms of vestibular migraine include vertigo in combination with headache, and these two symptoms often occur relatively close to each other[91]. Other symptoms can include transient hearing fluctuations[97], nausea, vomiting, and a sensitivity to motion sickness[95]. Some patients have reported triggering of their migraine in response to dehydration, lack of sleep, or certain foods, but the relationship between these characteristics and vestibular migraines has not been well-studied[95]. Evidence of effective treatment of vestibular migraines is limited. Patients who respond favorably to anti-migraine medication have occurred, but the evidence is lacking as to overall effectiveness[98].

Vestibular neuritis

Vestibular neuritis is associated with vertigo, nausea, vomiting, and imbalance, and is thought to be due to viral inflammation of the vestibular nerve[99]. The condition is acute in nature with symptoms lasting from a few days to several weeks, but up to half of those suffering from vestibular neuritis can experience symptoms much longer[100]. Vestibular neuritis has been reported to account for nearly 10% of all dizziness-related medical visits[101]. Interestingly, viral epidemics trigger an increased incidence of vestibular neuritis, lending evidence to its likely inflammatory origins[102].

Patients exhibiting vestibular neuritis will present with acute, severe vertigo[91]. The most severe attacks can last for one to two days and then gradually subside over the following weeks. Motion may worsen the vertigo, and some patients experience nausea and vomiting in conjunction with the vertigo[91]. Additional symptoms often include nystagmus along with a walking pattern in which the patient tends to lean toward the affected ear's side.

Treatment of vestibular neuritis includes symptomatic care along with vestibular rehabilitation, which can begin as soon as tolerable after cessation of immediate symptoms[91]. Vestibular rehabilitation has been reported to be successful when compared against no therapy[103]. If vestibular neuritis is severe, short-term hospitalization may be required[91].

Acoustic Neuroma

Acoustic neuromas, or 'vestibular schwannomas', are benign tumors[104] of the eighth (vestibulocochlear) nerve[105]. The tumor is slow-growing, but can interfere with other structures of the inner ear[106]. With an incidence of 1 in 100,000, acoustic neuromas are quite rare and mainly affect older adults[106]. The most common symptoms of acoustic neuroma include tinnitus as well as hearing loss in the affected ear[106]. Up to 15% of patients do not experience hearing loss or tinnitus but do report vertigo, and that vertigo often results in them tending to drift to one side.

Because they are rather slow-growing, treatment for an acoustic neuroma can range from conservative methods such as simple long-term observation to the more intensive use of radiation[107] and/or surgical removal[105, 108].

Concussion

Even a hit to the head has the potential to cause significant vestibular-related symptoms, and many of these symptoms mimic what one would expect from PPPD. Concussion is a type of traumatic brain injury that most often results from a direct hit to the head or a type of injury (e.g. whiplash) that causes the brain to move rapidly within the skull. Concussions are not uncommon, with over 3 million concussions thought to occur per year in the United States[109]. The cause of concussion can vary by age, as children and older adults most commonly experience concussion as a result of falls, while in adults the most common cause is motor vehicle accidents[110]. Athletic participation, especially high-contact sports such as football, hockey, or boxing is also a common cause for concussion and even includes a separate classification as *sport-related concussion*. Like many vestibular-related symptoms, imaging through x-ray, MRI, CT scan, etc. is relatively ineffective at diagnosing concussion. Therefore, diagnosis is typically reliant upon the patient's history, description of the event that caused the concussion, and their symptoms. The range of symptoms that can occur in response to concussion can vary but do have a close resemblance to many of the symptoms of PPPD. Typically, symptoms of concussion are classified into three areas – cognitive, emotional, and psychological. Cognitive symptoms include difficulty concentrating or thinking (i.e. 'brain fog') in addition to difficulty with information retention. Emotional symptoms of concussion can include irritability, sadness, or general nervousness. Physical symptoms probably have the most similarity to PPPD as they can include headache, blurry vision, nausea and/or vomiting, sensitivity to light or noise, and imbalance issues, among others[110]. With such similarity in symptoms between PPPD and concussion – particularly among athletes or those who are susceptible to head-trauma events – it is somewhat easy to understand how PPPD may initially be misinterpreted as a concussion event.

Treatment of concussion is generally successful at relieving the associated symptoms. One of the first lines of treatment for concussion is rest. This includes both cognitive rest such as avoiding or reducing tasks that require a significant amount of 'thinking' (e.g. homework, computer use, etc.) as well as physical rest that avoids strenuous activity. Avoidance of associated triggers such as bright lights and loud noise is also recommended[111].

One of the positive aspects of concussion is that, unlike many other vestibular conditions, proper treatment generally results in a full recovery. Some individuals do have extended symptoms (e.g. 3 or more months), but the majority of individuals who suffer a concussion have relief of symptoms in a week or less and are typically allowed to resume activity. Having a concussion can predispose an individual to having a future concussion, so care must be taken to limit the opportunity for future concussions to occur.

Conclusion

Few who have not experienced a vestibular disorder can understand the impact or frustration that it can cause. Being dizzy for a second or two because you stood up too fast is nowhere near as debilitating as ongoing vertigo, unsteadiness, or any other effects of a chronic vestibular condition. The unpredictability of the attacks and the helplessness that can result are at times overwhelming, in turn leaving the patient feeling isolated, depressed, and desperate for some sort of improvement.

Being one of the newest recognized conditions in the medical community can be a positive as well as a negative. On the one hand, the fact that PPPD is officially recognized as an independent medical condition is beneficial as it focuses attention on a particular condition and stimulates interest in curing or at least treating the condition. On the other hand, the short amount of time that PPPD has been officially recognized also means that there is not a strong background of medical research available which can be used to look for trends or patterns in the data that will help lead to beneficial treatments. Still, patients of PPPD can be encouraged by the fact that their medical condition now has an official identification. Instead of being told that *it's all in your head*, or to *just relax*, patients are now accepted as having a truly debilitating condition.

Despite the newness of PPPD as a medical condition, there is a good deal of research from which patients can be encouraged. Other related medical conditions such as *phobic postural vertigo* have provided a foundation of research into chronic dizziness. Now, with PPPD becoming more recognized as one of the leading causes of dizziness, researchers and medical professionals can use these previous findings to focus in on PPPD itself and hopefully improve treatment for those affected.

The intent of this book was to provide you a source of quality and up-to-date information into the relatively new world of PPPD. My hope is that I fulfilled this intent and was able to provide you a comprehensive yet understandable guide that expanded your understanding of PPPD. Given its young age as a medical condition, coupled with bits of information pulled from other related medical conditions (e.g. PPV), it was difficult at times to keep the book focused on PPPD. However, given that these other conditions are now grouped in with PPPD, it made perfect sense to use the information we have gained from investigating these other conditions and include the information in a book about PPPD.

As a patient of PPPD, you not doubt want answers and a cure now, after having lived for a significant amount of time with the miserable symptoms associated with PPPD. Unfortunately, the answers are not there yet. The encouraging thing, though, is that the answers are slowly arriving, one by one. One study may reveal something we didn't know before, while another outlines a particular treatment that does not work. We must be sure to take all of these findings into effect and continue to build on our body of knowledge that will eventually lead to effective treatment and maybe even a cure for PPPD.

Until then, I wish you the best of luck on your continued journey with PPPD.

Glossary

Acoustic neuroma: a benign tumor that grows on one of the nerves associated with the ear

Ampulla: a bulbous area of the semicircular canal that contains the cupula

Agoraphobia: an anxiety disorder that causes a fear of places or situations capable of inducing panic

Benign: not harmful

Benign paroxysmal positional vertigo: a condition of the inner ear thought to result from loose otoliths that can cause severe bouts of vertigo in response to certain head positions

Chronic subjective dizziness: a type of dizziness that brings about dizziness, lightheadedness, or unsteadiness, in absence of vertigo and with symptoms that often worsen in highly stimulating visual environments

Cochlea: the organ of the inner ear shaped like a snail's shell which is responsible for receiving vibrations from the eardrum and converting them into electrical signals for transmission to the brain

Cognitive behavioral therapy: a psycho-social intervention designed to change unfavorable actions and improve both a patient's symptoms and their emotional state

Concussion: an injury to the brain that results in temporary loss of normal brain function

Cupula: An organ that projects into the middle of each semicircular canal and detects fluid movement within the canal

Dizziness: a sensation of unsteadiness accompanied by a feeling of movement within the head

Endolymph: the potassium-rich fluid contained within the membranous labyrinth of the ear

Equilibrium: a state of overall balance

Hair Cell: sensory receptors located within the auditory and vestibular organs of the ear that transmit a signal to the brain in response to detection of head movement or sound vibrations

Incidence: the number of new cases of an illness in a particular time frame, such as a year

Inner Ear: the portion of the ear within the temporal bone that contains the semicircular canals and cochlea

Labyrinth: the portion of the ear containing the hearing and balance organs

Ménière's Disease: a condition of the inner ear comprised of symptoms that include vertigo, tinnitus, hearing loss, and the sensation of ear fullness

Middle Ear: the central cavity of the inner ear comprised of the empty space within the temporal bone located inside of the eardrum

Nystagmus: involuntary eye movement

Oscillopsia: a visual problem that causes objects within the field of vision to oscillate (move in small motions)

Otolith: a small crystalline structure of the inner ear that plays a role in balance and equilibrium

Outer Ear: That portion of the ear that is visible, along with the auditory canal

Pinna: the external portion of the ear

Phobic postural vertigo: an anxiety-related, chronic condition that brings about bursts of imbalance as well as short attacks of dizziness

Presbycusis: age-related hearing loss

Prevalence: the number of people who have a particular medical condition at one point in time

Resilience: the ability to recover quickly from difficulty or hardship

Saccule: A vertically-oriented organ embedded with otoliths that detects movement occurring in a vertical plane

Space and motion discomfort: a condition characterized by disorientation when in situations that exhibit moving visual patterns

Temporal bone: A bone that is positioned at the side and base of the skull which houses the vestibular and hearing organs

Utricle: a horizontally-oriented organ embedded with otoliths that detects movement occurring in a horizontal plane.

Vertigo: a sensation of spinning that is usually accompanied by a sudden loss of balance

Vestibular migraine: a condition consisting of attacks of migraine that may or may not include vestibular symptoms such as vertigo or dizziness

Vestibular nerve: the eighth cranial nerve, responsible for transmitting hearing and sensory information from the inner ear to the brain

Vestibular rehabilitation: an exercise program designed to target the vestibular system and improve balance, proprioception, and dizziness

Visual vertigo: Dizziness brought about by repetitive or moving objects within the field of vision

References

1. Ekdale, E.G., *Form and function of the mammalian inner ear.* Journal of anatomy, 2016. **228**(2): p. 324-337.
2. Schuknecht, H. and R. Ruby, *Cupulolithiasis*, in *Otophysiology.* 1973, Karger Publishers. p. 434-443.
3. Lawal, O. and D. Navaratnam, *Causes of Central Vertigo*, in *Diagnosis and Treatment of Vestibular Disorders.* 2019, Springer. p. 363-375.
4. Peng, B., *Cervical vertigo: historical reviews and advances.* World neurosurgery, 2018. **109**: p. 347-350.
5. Lee, A., *Diagnosing the cause of vertigo: a practical approach.* Hong Kong Med J, 2012. **18**(4): p. 327-32.
6. Glover, J.C., *Vestibular System*, in *Encyclopedia of Neuroscience*, L.R. Squire, Editor. 2004, Academic Press: Oxford. p. 127-132.
7. Florence, C.S., et al., *Medical costs of fatal and nonfatal falls in older adults.* Journal of the American Geriatrics Society, 2018. **66**(4): p. 693-698.
8. Whitman, G.T., *Dizziness.* The American journal of medicine, 2018. **131**(12): p. 1431-1437.
9. Muncie, H.L., S.M. Sirmans, and E. James, *Dizziness: Approach to Evaluation and Management.* American family physician, 2017. **95**(3): p. 154-162.
10. Neuhauser, H., et al., *Epidemiology of vestibular vertigo: a neurotologic survey of the general population.* Neurology, 2005. **65**(6): p. 898-904.
11. Tusa, R.J., *Dizziness.* Medical Clinics of North America, 2009. **93**(2): p. 263-271.
12. Neuhauser, H., *The epidemiology of dizziness and vertigo*, in *Handbook of clinical neurology.* 2016, Elsevier. p. 67-82.
13. Zamergrad, M., et al., *Common causes of vertigo and dizziness in different age groups of patients.* Bionanoscience, 2017. **7**(2): p. 259-262.
14. Lin, H.W. and N. Bhattacharyya, *Impact of dizziness and obesity on the prevalence of falls and fall-related injuries.* The Laryngoscope, 2014. **124**(12): p. 2797-2801.

15. Neuhauser, H.K., et al., *Burden of dizziness and vertigo in the community*. Archives of internal medicine, 2008. **168**(19): p. 2118-2124.
16. Whalley, M.G. and D.A. Cane, *A cognitive-behavioral model of persistent postural-perceptual dizziness*. Cognitive and Behavioral Practice, 2017. **24**(1): p. 72-89.
17. Ziegler, M.G. and R.R. Barager, *Postural hypotension and syncope*, in *Cardiovascular Disease in the Elderly*. 1993, Springer. p. 211-230.
18. Agrawal, Y., *Dizziness Demographics and Population Health*. Dizziness and Vertigo Across the Lifespan, 2018: p. 1.
19. Kesser, B.W. and A.T. Gleason, *Multisensory Imbalance and Presbystasis*, in *Diagnosis and Treatment of Vestibular Disorders*. 2019, Springer. p. 331-352.
20. Seemungal, B.M. and L. Passamonti, *Persistent postural-perceptual dizziness: a useful new syndrome*. 2018, BMJ Publishing Group Ltd.
21. Popkirov, S., J.P. Staab, and J. Stone, *Persistent postural-perceptual dizziness (PPPD): a common, characteristic and treatable cause of chronic dizziness*. Practical neurology, 2018. **18**(1): p. 5-13.
22. Bronstein, A., *Multisensory integration in balance control*, in *Handbook of clinical neurology*. 2016, Elsevier. p. 57-66.
23. Staab, J.P., *Functional and psychiatric vestibular disorders*, in *Handbook of clinical neurology*. 2016, Elsevier. p. 341-351.
24. Benedikt, M., *Über platzschwindel*. Allgemeine Wiener Medizinische Zeitung, 1870. **15**: p. 488-490.
25. Kuch, K. and R.P. Swinson, *Agoraphobia: what Westphal really said*. 1992, SAGE Publications Sage CA: Los Angeles, CA.
26. Lannois, M. and C. Tournier. *Les lesions auriculaires sont une cause determinante frequente de l'agoraphobie*. in *Annales des Maladies de L'oreille, du Larynx, du Nez et du Pharynx*. 1899.
27. Association, A.P., *Diagnostic and statistical manual of mental disorders*. BMC Med, 2013. **17**: p. 133-137.

28. Brandt, T. and M. Dieterich, *Phobischer attackenschwankschwindel, ein neues syndrom.* Münch Med Wochenschr, 1986. **128**: p. 247-250.
29. Jacob, R.G., et al., *Panic disorder with vestibular dysfunction: further clinical observations and description of space and motion phobic stimuli.* Journal of Anxiety Disorders, 1989. **3**(2): p. 117-130.
30. Bronstein, A.M., *Visual vertigo syndrome: clinical and posturography findings.* Journal of Neurology, Neurosurgery & Psychiatry, 1995. **59**(5): p. 472-476.
31. Pavlou, M., R.A. Davies, and A.M. Bronstein, *The assessment of increased sensitivity to visual stimuli in patients with chronic dizziness.* Journal of Vestibular Research, 2006. **16**(4, 5): p. 223-231.
32. Cousins, S., et al., *Visual dependency and dizziness after vestibular neuritis.* PLoS One, 2014. **9**(9): p. e105426.
33. Staab, J.P. and M.J. Ruckenstein, *Expanding the differential diagnosis of chronic dizziness.* Archives of Otolaryngology–Head & Neck Surgery, 2007. **133**(2): p. 170-176.
34. Dieterich, M., J.P. Staab, and T. Brandt, *Functional (psychogenic) dizziness,* in *Handbook of clinical neurology.* 2016, Elsevier. p. 447-468.
35. Staab, J.P., et al., *Diagnostic criteria for persistent postural-perceptual dizziness (PPPD): consensus document of the committee for the classification of vestibular disorders of the bárány society.* Journal of Vestibular Research, 2017. **27**(4): p. 191-208.
36. Nazareth, I., et al., *Outcome of symptoms of dizziness in a general practice community sample.* Family Practice, 1999. **16**(6): p. 616-618.
37. Staab, J.P., *Psychiatric Considerations in the Management of Dizzy Patients,* in *Vestibular Disorders.* 2019, Karger Publishers. p. 170-179.
38. Yan, Z., et al., *Analysis of the characteristics of persistent postural-perceptual dizziness: A clinical-based study in China.* International journal of audiology, 2017. **56**(1): p. 33-37.
39. Yagi, C., et al., *A Validated Questionnaire to Assess the Severity of Persistent Postural-Perceptual Dizziness*

(PPPD): *The Niigata PPPD Questionnaire (NPQ).* Otology & Neurotology, 2019.

40. Staab, J.P., *Chronic subjective dizziness.* CONTINUUM: Lifelong Learning in Neurology, 2012. **18**(5): p. 1118-1141.

41. Trinidade, A. and J.A. Goebel, *Persistent Postural-Perceptual Dizziness—A Systematic Review of the Literature for the Balance Specialist.* Otology & Neurotology, 2018. **39**(10): p. 1291-1303.

42. Holle, D., et al., *Persistent postural-perceptual dizziness: a matter of higher, central dysfunction?* PLoS One, 2015. **10**(11): p. e0142468.

43. Adamec, I., et al., *O-01 Persistent postural-perceptual dizziness: clinical and neurophysiological study.* Clinical Neurophysiology, 2019. **130**(7): p. e21.

44. Riccelli, R., et al., *Altered insular and occipital responses to simulated vertical self-motion in patients with persistent postural-perceptual dizziness.* Frontiers in neurology, 2017. **8**: p. 529.

45. Wurthmann, S., et al., *Cerebral gray matter changes in persistent postural perceptual dizziness.* Journal of psychosomatic research, 2017. **103**: p. 95-101.

46. Na, S., et al., *Cerebral perfusion abnormalities in patients with persistent postural-perceptual dizziness (PPPD): a SPECT study.* Journal of Neural Transmission, 2019. **126**(2): p. 123-129.

47. Lee, J.O., et al., *Altered brain function in persistent postural perceptual dizziness: A study on resting state functional connectivity.* Human brain mapping, 2018. **39**(8): p. 3340-3353.

48. Van Ombergen, A., et al., *Altered functional brain connectivity in patients with visually induced dizziness.* NeuroImage: Clinical, 2017. **14**: p. 538-545.

49. Kapfhammer, H., et al., *Course of illness in phobic postural vertigo.* Acta neurologica scandinavica, 1997. **95**(1): p. 23-28.

50. Tschan, R., et al., *Patients' psychological well-being and resilient coping protect from secondary somatoform vertigo and dizziness (SVD) 1 year after vestibular disease.* Journal of neurology, 2011. **258**(1): p. 104-112.

51.   Best, C., et al., *Who is at risk for ongoing dizziness and psychological strain after a vestibular disorder?* Neuroscience, 2009. **164**(4): p. 1579-1587.
52.   Staab, J.P., et al., *Anxious, introverted personality traits in patients with chronic subjective dizziness.* Journal of psychosomatic research, 2014. **76**(1): p. 80-83.
53.   Beck, A. and G. Emery. *with Greenberg, RL (1985). Anxiety disorders and phobias: A cognitive perspective.* in *Library of congress, USA.* 1973.
54.   Whitman, G.T., *Examination of the Patient with Dizziness or Imbalance.* Medical Clinics, 2019. **103**(2): p. 191-201.
55.   Cheng, H.M., J.H. Park, and D. Hernstadt, *Subacute combined degeneration of the spinal cord following recreational nitrous oxide use.* BMJ case reports, 2013. **2013**: p. bcr2012008509.
56.   Findlay, G.F., et al., *Does walking change the Romberg sign?* European spine journal, 2009. **18**(10): p. 1528-1531.
57.   Söhsten, E., R.S. Bittar, and J.P. Staab, *Posturographic profile of patients with persistent postural-perceptual dizziness on the sensory organization test.* Journal of Vestibular Research, 2016. **26**(3): p. 319-326.
58.   Popkirov, S., J. Stone, and D. Holle-Lee, *Treatment of Persistent Postural-Perceptual Dizziness (PPPD) and Related Disorders.* Current treatment options in neurology, 2018. **20**(12): p. 50.
59.   Badke, M.B., et al., *Effects of vestibular and balance rehabilitation on sensory organization and dizziness handicap.* Annals of Otology, Rhinology & Laryngology, 2005. **114**(1): p. 48-54.
60.   Staab, J.P., *Behavioral aspects of vestibular rehabilitation.* NeuroRehabilitation, 2011. **29**(2): p. 179-183.
61.   Thompson, K.J., et al., *Retrospective review and telephone follow-up to evaluate a physical therapy protocol for treating persistent postural-perceptual dizziness: a pilot study.* Journal of Vestibular Research, 2015. **25**(2): p. 97-104.
62.   Edelman, S., A.E. Mahoney, and P.D. Cremer, *Cognitive behavior therapy for chronic subjective*

dizziness: a randomized, controlled trial. American journal of otolaryngology, 2012. **33**(4): p. 395-401.
63. Brandt, T., D. Huppert, and M. Dieterich, *Phobic postural vertigo: a first follow-up.* Journal of neurology, 1994. **241**(4): p. 191-195.
64. Holmberg, J., et al., *Treatment of phobic postural vertigo.* Journal of neurology, 2006. **253**(4): p. 500-506.
65. Holmberg, J., et al., *One-year follow-up of cognitive behavioral therapy for phobic postural vertigo.* Journal of neurology, 2007. **254**(9): p. 1189.
66. Goto, F., T. Tsutsumi, and K. Ogawa, *Treatment of chronic subjective dizziness by SSRIs.* Nihon Jibiinkoka Gakkai Kaiho, 2013. **116**(11): p. 1208-1213.
67. Yu, Y.-C., et al., *Cognitive behavior therapy as augmentation for sertraline in treating patients with persistent postural-perceptual dizziness.* BioMed research international, 2018. **2018**.
68. Rascol, O., et al., *Antivertigo medications and drug-induced vertigo.* Drugs, 1995. **50**(5): p. 777-791.
69. Aaronson, S.T., et al., *A 5-year observational study of patients with treatment-resistant depression treated with vagus nerve stimulation or treatment as usual: comparison of response, remission, and suicidality.* American Journal of Psychiatry, 2017. **174**(7): p. 640-648.
70. Gaul, C., et al. *gammaCore (R) use for prevention and acute treatment of chronic cluster headache: findings from the randomized phase of the PREVA study.* in *ANNALS OF NEUROLOGY.* 2014. WILEY-BLACKWELL 111 RIVER ST, HOBOKEN 07030-5774, NJ USA.
71. Eren, O.E., et al., *Non-invasive vagus nerve stimulation significantly improves quality of life in patients with persistent postural-perceptual dizziness.* Journal of neurology, 2018. **265**(1): p. 63-69.
72. Palm, U., et al., *Transcranial direct current stimulation (tDCS) for treatment of phobic postural vertigo: an open label pilot study.* European archives of psychiatry and clinical neuroscience, 2019. **269**(2): p. 269-272.
73. Bronstein, A.M., *Vision and vertigo.* Journal of neurology, 2004. **251**(4): p. 381-387.

74. Witkin, H.A. and S.E. Asch, *Studies in space orientation. IV. Further experiments on perception of the upright with displaced visual fields.* Journal of experimental psychology, 1948. **38**(6): p. 762.

75. Page, N. and M.A. Gresty, *Motorist's vestibular disorientation syndrome.* Journal of Neurology, Neurosurgery & Psychiatry, 1985. **48**(8): p. 729-735.

76. Guerraz, M., et al., *Visual vertigo: symptom assessment, spatial orientation and postural control.* Brain, 2001. **124**(8): p. 1646-1656.

77. Ketola, S., et al., *Somatoform disorders in vertiginous children and adolescents.* International journal of pediatric otorhinolaryngology, 2009. **73**(7): p. 933-936.

78. Obermann, M., et al., *Long-term outcome of vertigo and dizziness associated disorders following treatment in specialized tertiary care: the Dizziness and Vertigo Registry (DiVeR) Study.* Journal of neurology, 2015. **262**(9): p. 2083-2091.

79. Brandt, T., et al., *Artificial neural network posturography detects the transition of vestibular neuritis to phobic postural vertigo.* Journal of neurology, 2012. **259**(1): p. 182-184.

80. Wuehr, M., et al., *Inadequate interaction between open- and closed-loop postural control in phobic postural vertigo.* Journal of neurology, 2013. **260**(5): p. 1314-1323.

81. Huppert, D., T. Kunihiro, and T. Brandt, *Phobic postural vertigo (154 patients): its association with vestibular disorders.* Journal of Audiological Medicine, 1995. **4**(2): p. 97-103.

82. Dieterich, M., M. Obermann, and N. Celebisoy, *Vestibular migraine: the most frequent entity of episodic vertigo.* Journal of neurology, 2016. **263**(1): p. 82-89.

83. Minor, L.B., D.A. Schessel, and J.P. Carey, *Ménière's disease.* Current opinion in neurology, 2004. **17**(1): p. 9-16.

84. Ishiyama, G., I. Lopez, and A. Ishiyama, *Aquaporins and Ménière's disease.* Current Opinion in Otolaryngology & Head and Neck Surgery, 2006. **14**(5): p. 332-336.

85. Rauch, S.D., *Clinical Hints and Precipitating Factors in Patients Suffering from Ménière's Disease.* Otolaryngologic Clinics of North America, 2010. **43**(5): p. 1011-1017.

86. Kangasniemi, E. and E. Hietikko, *The theory of autoimmunity in Ménière's disease is lacking evidence.* Auris Nasus Larynx, 2018. **45**(3): p. 399-406.

87. Vrabec, J.T., *Herpes simplex virus and Ménière's Disease.* The Laryngoscope, 2003. **113**(9): p. 1431-1438.

88. Bjorne, A., A. Berven, and G. Agerberg, *Cervical Signs and Symptoms in Patients with Ménière's Disease: A Controlled Study.* CRANIO®, 1998. **16**(3): p. 194-202.

89. Soderman, A.C.H., et al., *Stress as a Trigger of Attacks in Menière's Disease. A Case-Crossover Study.* The Laryngoscope, 2004. **114**(10): p. 1843-1848.

90. Hanley, K., *Symptoms of vertigo in general practice: a prospective study of diagnosis.* Br J Gen Pract, 2002. **52**(483): p. 809-812.

91. Wipperman, J., *Dizziness and vertigo.* Primary Care: Clinics in Office Practice, 2014. **41**(1): p. 115-131.

92. Bhattacharyya, N., et al., *Clinical practice guideline: benign paroxysmal positional vertigo.* Otolaryngology--Head and Neck Surgery, 2008. **139**(5_suppl): p. 47-81.

93. Cherchi, M. and T.C. Hain, *Migraine-associated vertigo.* Otolaryngologic Clinics of North America, 2011. **44**(2): p. 367-375.

94. Neuhauser, H., et al., *Migrainous vertigo Prevalence and impact on quality of life.* Neurology, 2006. **67**(6): p. 1028-1033.

95. Lempert, T., et al., *Vestibular migraine: diagnostic criteria.* Journal of Vestibular Research, 2012. **22**(4): p. 167-172.

96. Abu-Arafeh, I. and G. Russell, *Paroxysmal vertigo as a migraine equivalent in children: a population-based study.* Cephalalgia, 1995. **15**(1): p. 22-25.

97. Johnson, G.D., *Medical management of migraine-related dizziness and vertigo.* The Laryngoscope, 1998. **108**(S85): p. 1-28.

98. Fotuhi, M., et al., *Vestibular migraine: a critical review of treatment trials.* Journal of neurology, 2009. **256**(5): p. 711-716.

99. Schuknecht, H.F. and K. Kitamura, *Vestibular neuritis.* Annals of Otology, Rhinology & Laryngology, 1981. **90**(1_suppl): p. 1-19.

100. Perols, J.B., Olle, *Vestibular neuritis: a follow-up study.* Acta oto-laryngologica, 1999. **119**(8): p. 895-899.

101. Neuhauser, H.K. and T. Lempert. *Vertigo: epidemiologic aspects.* in *Seminars in neurology.* 2009. © Thieme Medical Publishers.

102. Baloh, R.W. and V. Honrubia, *Clinical neurophysiology of the vestibular system.* 2001: Oxford University Press, USA.

103. Hillier, S.L. and M. McDonnell, *Vestibular rehabilitation for unilateral peripheral vestibular dysfunction.* The Cochrane Library, 2011.

104. Nikolopoulos, T.P., et al., *Acoustic Neuroma Growth: A Systematic Review of the Evidence.* Otology & Neurotology, 2010. **31**(3): p. 478-485.

105. McLaughlin, E.J., et al., *Quality of Life in Acoustic Neuroma Patients.* Otology & Neurotology, 2015. **36**(4): p. 653-656.

106. Rosahl, S., et al., *Diagnostics and therapy of vestibular schwannomas–an interdisciplinary challenge.* GMS current topics in otorhinolaryngology, head and neck surgery, 2017. **16**.

107. McClelland, S.I., et al., *Impact of Race and Insurance Status on Surgical Approach for Cervical Spondylotic Myelopathy in the United States: A Population-Based Analysis.* Spine, 2017. **42**(3): p. 186-194.

108. Fusco, M.R., et al., *Current practices in vestibular schwannoma management: A survey of American and Canadian neurosurgeons.* Clinical Neurology and Neurosurgery, 2014. **127**: p. 143-148.

109. Brain Injury Research Institute. *What is a concussion?* ; Available from: http://www.protectthebrain.org/.

110. Centers for Disease Control and Prevention, *Traumatic Brain Injury and Concussion.* 2019.

111. Broglio, S.P., et al., *National Athletic Trainers' Association position statement: management of sport*

concussion. Journal of athletic training, 2014. **49**(2): p. 245-265.

Let others know!

If you found this or any of Mark's other books informative, *please take the time and post a review online!* Reviews help get exposure for the books and thereby improve the chances that others will be able to benefit from the material as well.

Check out these other books by Mark Knoblauch

Challenge the Hand You Were Dealt: Strategies to battle back against adversity and improve your chances for success

Essentials of Writing and Publishing Your Self-Help Book

Living Low Sodium: A guide for understanding our relationship with sodium and how to be successful in adhering to a low-sodium diet

Outlining Tinnitus: A comprehensive guide to help you break free of the ringing in your ears

Overcoming Ménière's: How changing your lifestyle can change your life

Professional Writing in Kinesiology and Sports Medicine

Seven Ways To Make Running Not Suck

The Art of Efficiency: A guide for improving task management in the home to help maximize your leisure time

Understanding BPPV: Outlining the causes and effects of Benign Paroxysmal Positional Vertigo

Vestibular Migraine: A Comprehensive Patient Guide

A Patient's Guide to Acoustic Neuroma

Vestibular Migraine – Patient Logbook

About the Author

Mark is a small-town Kansas native who now lives in a suburb of Houston with his wife and two young daughters. His background is in the area of sports medicine, obtaining his bachelor's degree from Wichita State and his master's degree from the University of Nevada, Las Vegas. After working clinically as an athletic trainer for eight years, Mark returned to graduate school where he received his doctorate in Kinesiology from the University of Houston, followed by a postdoctoral assistantship in Molecular Physiology and Biophysics at Baylor College of Medicine in Houston, TX. He has been employed as a college professor at the University of Houston since 2013.

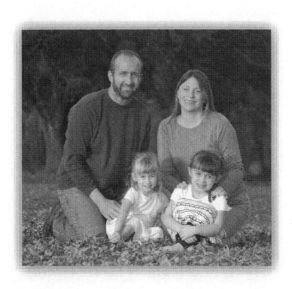

Image Credits:

Image 1.1: shutterstock.com/Medical Art Inc
Image 1.2: shutterstock.com/ilusmedical
Image 1.3: shutterstock.com/maxcreatnz
Image 1.4: shutterstock.com/Designua
Image 1.5: shutterstock.com/Designua

Front Cover Image: shutterstock.com/Andrus Ciprian

Printed in Great Britain
by Amazon

49491684R00079